to Vic

Healing
the
Wounds
of War

Best wishes!

outskirts
press

Dear brother, Amnon,

I am overwhelmed. I just saw your film once again and read your book once more, this time in its entirety. You brought me to a state of being with a perspective on life that, in these trying times, all but eludes me. Next to what you shared in your narrative, one that allowed me to feel and live through the most intimate encounter I've ever had with war, with the internal suffering and struggle of someone who all but died in battle, who ultimately survived, rescued by those who knew they were inviting death by attempting to do so — ultimately a triumph of love over darkness and despair — makes the world around me reveal itself to be, in many ways, superficial, devoid of the depth of life, pain, courage and real love that you have shared in your book and film, "I Will Not Forget This, My Friend". I am different now, clear and transformed by this moment. Through you, I've touched the truth of what life is, in a way I've never encountered before. Life is suffering and love, woven into each other, in ways that are so sad and deep, that they are only equaled by the music of your song, with its extraordinary lyrics by the poet Nathan Alterman, I knew this song was extraordinary when I first heard it. Now I know why. For me, it is a cry to the world to embrace and heal our collective sorrow, our wounded souls, and a cry to all of us to transform that sorrow into love. Such transformation, I believe, is the only way to heal the depth of pain and loss that you have experienced and shared in your book, your film and your music — and is the only pathway for all of us to follow if we are to be able to carry on in life to somehow survive, preserve our humanity, and ultimately allow the beauty of life to shine once more upon us.

Love,
Peter Yarrow
(of Peter, Paul & Mary)

5/18/18

Dear Amnon,

Thank you for sharing your manuscript with me along with the video.

First let me say the video is extraordinarily powerful and anyone seeing, and for those whose heritage is in Israel, I'm sure it is a compelling commemoration of a landmark event in the nation's history. I am privileged to have seen it. Thank you. (It was also a special surprise to hear Steve Hubbard as the "voice over)

Your manuscript is an impressive piece of writing. You convey vividly how the battle at the Nebbi Yusha fortress, and the casualty you received there, shaped your journey for the rest of your life. You are a good writer, able with restrained prose to articulate that journey of coming to terms with both the physical and emotional scars war left on you. In the end your tale is an heroic one of a man who, thrown into the chaos of war so young and vulnerable, comes to find peace.

If you will allow me, "I will not forget this, my friend."

Reverend Mark Trotter,
Retired, United Methodist Minister
San Diego, California

I needed to read the book again; then I was moved to read it once more.

Thanks for writing this very personal story. I was moved by the sincerity contained in your writings. For those of us who have had to ask the question - why me? - You unlocked the answer in the last sentence of your book. LOVE.

I believe your story will have an impact far greater than just writing a book. It carries a message. That message is always LOVE, love of your fellow man.

The tempo and sincerity of your story is a message that will assist others to better understand their responsibility and role in this world. For many, your story will bring peace in their personal life. We owe you a great debt for your courage and inspiration.

Thank you my brother.

Your Friend,
Larry Scott
San Diego, California

""Healing the Wounds of War" is an amazing story and one that should be told. The tragic and ill-fated battle of Nebbi Yusha, as told by Amnon in this book, is tremendously moving and riveting. It holds a bold symbolism that parallels Amnon's own remarkable life and reminds us to be a witness to truth while giving honor to those who have touched or helped us and even sacrificed their own lives - whether literally or figuratively - for the betterment of others. It's a story of the indomitable pluck of the human spirit and the will to persevere and triumph even when the odds are against you. Amnon's life inspires us to seek more and never settle."

Wishing you all the best, always.

Warm hugs and love,
Alyssa Martina

Dedication

This book is dedicated to the many who saved my life under the most arduous conditions, and to my wife Selma Lee who has been by my side all these years.

Table of Contents

III. THE CRISIS

IV. THE REWARDS

Introduction

This book has been very difficult to write because of its very painful and sensitive subject. Several attempts over the years have ended with either one story that I filed away or nothing at all.

It took me forty years of suffering in silence before a crisis forced me to confront my ghosts and devils. It was only then that I began to consider the idea of possibly writing a book.

I am deeply indebted to cousins Jim and Randy Weiss who invited me in October 2016 to their home in Virginia for the purpose of recording my book in their professional studio, under Jim's able guidance. I came prepared with an outline and we worked some two hours a day for seven days. A preliminary rough draft was born.

I had a very clear purpose for writing this book -- being eager to share my healing journey with other combat soldiers, regardless of which war they served in, who were still struggling secretly in silence with their demons. In many ways we are all brothers.

I also felt my book could provide the general public an insight into the psyche of those who come home from a combat experience.

I.
THE WAR

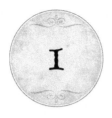

Awakening

"I'm awake ... clear mind ... I'M ALIVE!!! ... I'M SAFE! ... I DID NOT DIE.... "

"Where am I? ... How did I get here? ... How long has it been? ... I am so weak, I am falling asleep ... sleep ... sleep ...."

———⟊⟊⟊———

Thoughts were flashing in my mind ... I was flat on my back ... the soft bed was so comfortable ...it was quiet ... I was so weak and tired ... just wanted to sleep ... happy to be alive! ... sleep ... sleep ...

———⟊⟊⟊———

Something was pressing hard against my rib cage on my right ... what was it? ... A foreign object in my bed? ... Sleep ... sleep ...sleep ... I was so tired...

———◦◦◦◦◦———

I remembered the battle ... how did it end? ... We were in retreat ... I was firing at the fortress ... a powerful blow hit my head ... a bullet! ... a black curtain in front of my eyes ... I was floating like a feather in a dark space ... the air was coming out of my lungs ... I felt very cold ... quiet ... total helplessness ... I knew I was dying ... I felt comfortable ... in my mind I thought, "Farewell Father, Mother, friends..." and the dark black curtain took over ...

———◦◦◦◦◦———

I was screaming ... the smell of ether was so powerful ... they were changing the dressing on my head ... the head felt so cold ... sleep ... sleep ... I was so tired ...

It was timeless ... I'd wake up between long sleep periods ... flat on my back in bed ... I was so weak and very comfortable ...

"Aha, I survived! ... Was my brain intact? ... a terrifying thought ... and what damage to other body parts...?"

"How did the battle end? ... Any casualties? ... what did happen on the north side...?"

I tested myself in my mind... I used to be good in math ...

"$(A + B)^2 = A^2 + 2AB + B^2$ . . . I am OK! - I am OK! - MY BRAIN IS OK! ... I will survive ... I'm so weak and tired now ...sleep ... sleep...."

Next I was waiting for my first erection, being assured I was still a man.

———

"I will fully recover, I know it ... my mind is clear. I will overcome the weakness ... I will eat and exercise my way to health ... but my right arm ... it's so weak, I can hardly lift it ... as if it was not connected to my body... sleep ... sleep...."

———

I opened my eyes. My young sister Erela's face was about one foot above mine. She had been trying to wake me up, get my attention.

I was so happy to see her! But I could not move, I was so tired. Her famous beauty spot was still on her nose. I muttered the familiar Yiddish phrase: "Pintale Nosell." And she replied with her favorite call: "Hello,

Bro." I could vaguely see my parents standing behind her. I was falling into a deep sleep again.

For the following week or so, I was still barely able to speak. I did hear the words in my head but was unable to process them through my mouth. I was terribly frustrated and extremely tired.

⚊⊸⊸⊱⟊⟊⊰⊷⊷⚊

I was hearing piano music coming from the outside through the open balcony door. A familiar Chopin nocturne. It was as if I were hearing music for the first time in my life. It was so rich and beautiful, a powerful reintroduction to life's beauty. I was overcome with emotions and began to cry with joy. It was so good to be alive! Memories were being reawakened.

⚊⊸⊸⊱⟊⟊⊰⊷⊷⚊

Two male orderlies were cleaning the room and making the beds. In the background I heared the sound of music, perhaps from a radio, recognizing it as "The Moldau" by Smetana. Listening to the music awakened wonderful memories from the past and spoke to my soul.

The two orderlies were arguing who the composer was - - "Tchaikovsky -- no -- Schubert" --- and so they went, back and forth, while I was trying with all my might to tell them how wrong they were.

I was still in the period when I could not process thoughts into words through my mouth.

My body was shaking with frustration. Suddenly, out of nowhere, I burst out: "SMETANA!" – to their great shock.

⟶⟶⟶

My right arm was so heavy! My right hand was "useless": no feeling and no strength. It was my right arm pressing against my rib cage that earlier felt like a foreign object in bed.

⟶⟶⟶

Several days after surgery, I began to spend more time awake between long periods of sleep. I was hungry. I was famished. I kept asking for more food. Later on, when I could get out of bed by myself, I was allowed to enter the kitchen at will to get more food. I was being treated like a prince, or the miracle man coming back from the dead.

⟶⟶⟶

Two nurses were supporting me on my first walk out of bed, perhaps some ten days after surgery. I slowly stepped towards the door to the balcony. Up to that time, life was in a "black and white" world; the walls, ceiling, bed sheets, nurses' uniforms, were all white. Stepping to the balcony, I was overwhelmed by the symphony of colors, particularly the rich green of the lawn directly in front. Tears filled my eyes. I was catching up with nature's beauty, reawakening my memory.

—⚬—

I loved each and every nurse who cared for me. They were so caring, pleasant, and helpful. They were amazing.

—⚬—

Once I could get out of bed by myself, and speech was back although a bit slow, I visited the main ward to introduce myself. I didn't realize I was famous -- many cheered for me. They used to hear me screaming as the doctor was changing the dressing on my head -- I was actually shouting battlefield commands as if I were still out there. The screaming stopped once I snapped out of my coma. I began to socialize with other wounded soldiers on our floor. I visited the kitchen often: I couldn't eat enough. I was also pumped with penicillin. I spent time on the balcony soaking in the warm spring sun, feeling good and happy to be alive. My good old happy youthful spirits were coming back.

—⚬—

Two old friends visited me at the hospital. Ditza was my former high school girlfriend; Miriam was the girlfriend of a close friend. They gently told me the bad news. The battle ended in utter disaster. We lost a total of twenty-two men from a force of eighty; twelve were from our own Daphna group. They gently doled out their names, one at a time, as I was slipping into shock and utter disbelief; they were the best of the best, some also childhood friends of mine.

Also lost was our platoon commander, my direct commander, "Dudu," who went on to become a heroic mythological figure.

I was unequipped to handle the terrible news. I was shocked; I wanted to cry, but didn't dare. I put on a stone face, pretending I was strong and unaffected, but deep inside I was crushed, sad, angry, empty, and confused. I got into a protective shell that lasted some forty years.

I was very happy to have survived but was unable to express and enjoy it, as if that would be disloyal to those who perished and to their loved ones. The guilt of survival would haunt me for decades to come: "Why me and not them?" I felt helplessly trapped in between, showing only a stone face.

I began to realize my survival was a true miracle. The bullet went through my head, entering over the left ear and somehow missing the brain. The damage was due to blood pressing on the brain, causing paralysis of the right hand and short-term loss of sight and speech. Fortunately, the blood clotted and did not penetrate the brain. Through extensive rehab, the paralysis ultimately morphed into a condition called stereognosis of the right hand, meaning I am unable to identify or discern objects or textures with the right hand and fingers, nor do I know where the hand and fingers are without looking at them.

The battle took place near Israel's northern border with Lebanon, a place called Nebbi Yusha. My injury occurred at about 4:00 a.m. on Tuesday and I immediately fell into a coma that lasted some eight days. I did not receive significant medical treatment for 72 hours until I arrived at the Beilinson hospital in central Israel on Thursday evening or Friday morning.

I knew I was rescued from the battlefield by my comrades but had no idea how I arrived at the hospital near Tel-Aviv 72 hours later. I had to wait forty years before I began to put the story together.

I was operated on by Dr. Harden Askenasy, at the time one of the world's foremost neurosurgeons, who had arrived in Israel from the Cyprus refugee detention camp some two weeks earlier as a Holocaust survivor from Romania. I was the first or one of his first soldier patients. He removed a 4X4" part of my skull over the left ear to relieve pressure from the brain. Following surgery, he gave me a 0.5% chance of making it.

I fooled them all. I recovered from loss of sight and speech in short order, but I permanently lost the feelings and control of the right hand, my dominant one.

—⁂—

The survival miracle was not occupying my mind at that time. I was focused on whatever it took to return to normal healthy life, even returning to my military unit. I was feeling reborn, with life's great opportunities ahead. Healing my body and brainpower were highest on my list of priorities. The emotional component was totally avoided and not being attended to, as if it did not exist.

—⁂—

I had great confidence in Dr. Askenasy. His eyes and mannerisms exuded confidence, empathy, and authority. A newcomer to the country, he did not speak Hebrew, so I resorted to my high school English. He became my second father, a lifelong relationship. I knew my recovery made him feel so proud.

—⁂—

The hospital was overloaded with wounded soldiers, and extra beds crowded the hallways. Seventeen days after admission I was released from the hospital for one month in a convalescent center. I asked to first go home. I was eager to go home after eight months' absence; home with Mom's care and cooking, Father's calm strength and support, back to my roots and secure place. I was exactly eighteen years and four months old.

After one week at home I was ready to go to the convalescent center for a month. That was around 15th of May 1948, when Israel officially declared itself a state and the British evacuated the land.

We stayed in a fairly new building, two to a large room, and were well fed and cared for. There was a clubroom with board games, and that was about it. I was very weak, very much under the head injury trauma, and unable to use my right hand. I also had a 4"X4" soft area over the left ear where a part of the skull had been removed in surgery. I was just happy to be in my own quiet place and not do much. I was feeling weak, numb, remote, and introspective.

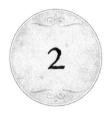

Palmach and Me

Palmach is an acronym in Hebrew for Shock Troops. It was the active striking force of the Haganah (meaning "defense" in Hebrew) Jewish underground during the British occupation of Palestine. The Haganah was formed to provide security for Jewish communities against Arab terrorist attacks, and it was subordinated to the main Jewish political authorities.

It was customary for high school graduates in the mid-1940s to volunteer for one-year community service for the greater cause. Many served as instructors in the underground Haganah. The epitome of service was a two-year full-time commitment to the Palmach.

Platoon-sized units were stationed in a kibbutz and supported themselves by working at the kibbutz half the time; the other half was dedicated to military training. To the outside world members appeared like farm workers. Following the Second World War, Palmach units were at the forefront of resistance against the British in Palestine and also ran the campaign of bringing ships with holocaust survivors from Europe to the Promised Land, trying to break the British blockade.

Following the two-year service, members became part of the active reserve, on call for underground operations.

Our group consisted of scout movement troops from Tel Aviv, Haifa and Jerusalem, totaling some seventy-five young men and thirty-five young women. Joining the Palmach upon high school graduation was a natural step for us; following the two-year service, we would proceed to form a new kibbutz of our own. Settling the land was the pioneering call of the time.

We were a rather homogenous group, generally native-born with parents arriving from Eastern Europe in the early 1920s. Most of us were high school graduates, usually good students, the best of the best.

My father arrived in Palestine as a pioneer in 1920 from a small town in Poland and settled in Tel-Aviv. My mother, his childhood sweetheart, followed him in 1925. My older brother was born in 1927, and I was born in 1929. My sister was born five years later. When I was six, we moved into a new apartment in a building built by my father; it would become my permanent home through adulthood. In childhood we did not have many luxuries, but life was full, safe, and comfortable. At age six I joined the Cub Scouts and also began taking violin lessons. At age twelve, I joined the Sea Scouts, and at thirteen I joined the youth part of the Haganah underground.

Public elementary school was of excellent quality, with fine teachers and valuable discipline. In addition to major subjects we had arts and crafts, gardening, chorus, band, orchestra, and athletics. We started English classes in the fifth grade. There were no social promotions. Passing final exams was required to proceed to high school. In high school, I played the violin in the orchestra when we produced and gave ten performances of the opera *Aida* by Verdi. To graduate from high school required passing all six national standard final exams on major subjects. Based on my high school diploma alone I was later admitted directly as a sophomore to U.C. Berkeley, one of the top public universities in the USA. This was standard, not the exception.

Being a member of the Haganah underground left its mark on me. Both my older brother and father were members as well, in different units, and we never talked about it at home. The less I knew, the safer it was. No police could pry from me information I did not know. I learned to be careful how I communicated. We also learned to show no emotions, keep a "stiff upper lip."

My activities in the Haganah began with training in self-defense techniques, open field training, and use of a handgun. We were used as message carriers for higher-ups and spotters against the British. Several times I was a messenger for my own father. As a young teenager, I dreamed of the time after high school when I would join the elite Palmach unit and see real action.

A life-altering event happened to me around 1943/4 when I was about thirteen years old. My parents and I were listening to a special radio broadcast listing names of Jewish communities in Poland that had been decimated by the Germans in the Holocaust. When the name of my parents' hometown was announced, they both broke down crying. I was deeply moved, cried with them, and "never again" was deeply etched into my DNA; this will never happen to us here! We will fight and resist to the last drop of blood!

Starting when I was twelve, we would spend parts of summer vacations on a kibbutz, providing helping hands during the active summer season. We'd go as an organized high school class with a teacher, or as a scout troop. I also attended underground training camps. Life was busy, purposeful, and exciting.

Two summers in a row I attended seamanship-training camps sponsored by the Jewish Agency. I graduated from the second one with top marks. Following WWII, graduates would serve as crews on ships bringing "illegal" Jewish refugees from Europe to the Promised Land, while trying to break the British blockade.

June 16,1946, was a historic date. The British conducted a country-wide campaign aimed at arresting the Haganah leadership and Palmach members. Our high school class with its teacher were spending a month at that time working in a kibbutz. We woke up early in the morning of the 16th with the kibbutz being surrounded by British troops who began a search for the Palmach unit stationed there. No luck; that unit had slipped out the night before. Our class was mistakenly identified as the Palmach unit, and we ended up spending a week in a detention camp in Atlit.

High school graduation in 1947 could not come soon enough for me. I was eager to join the Palmach and see real action. I had a choice between the Palmach marine unit, becoming involved with the "illegal" immigration of Holocaust survivors to the Promised Land, and the regular Palmach together with my many friends from the scout troops and high school. I chose the latter based on social considerations -- we were a happy social group of teenage boys and girls.

We spent the entire summer of 1947 working in three adjacent kibbutzim, getting acquainted and integrating into a cohesive social unit.

In September 1947 we arrived about 110 strong, 75 men and 35 women, at kibbutz Daphna in Northern Galilee, close to the Lebanese and Syrian borders. It was going to be our home for the next two years. We moved into long tin huts, each divided by jute partitions into four tiny rooms, each large enough to hold four beds against the walls. We also had a clubroom for community and social activities.

We did a lot of community singing and dancing, mainly waltzes, polkas, and the tango. Two members played the accordion, one was a fine pianist, and I had my violin.

Our time was split between work and military training. The job I detested most was the night guard shift; I had a very hard time staying awake the entire eight-hour shift. The one I enjoyed the most was waiting in the general dining hall.

I had no idea at the time how fast things were going to change! I was not prepared emotionally, and it took me some time to adjust.

The big change came around the middle of November, in anticipation of the United Nations' vote on the 29th for the creation of a State of Israel. In anticipation of Arab hostilities there was a need to rapidly expand the ranks of our underground military trained people. I was among fourteen of our own young men ordered into a special accelerated training camp and then to the Palmach squad command-training course. It meant the end of life in Daphna as we knew it, because upon graduation we would be assigned as squad leaders to other Palmach units elsewhere around the country. I hated the thought of being torn away from my life in Daphna and decided to do all I could to avoid it. I fabricated a medical excuse and managed to be released. I thought I was good and loyal to the cause, but actually I was unaware of the great historic changes coming upon us!

We entered the war footing in Daphna, and our lives took a drastic change. We stopped working in the kibbutz and began full-time intensive training. War was on the horizon and we were now full-time soldiers. It was an awkward period, since the British were still governing the country, and our arms were "illegal."

The War

With Arab hostilities upon us, our arms were coming out of hiding -- British army rifles, Bren light machine guns, Sten sub-machine guns, grenades, and 2" and 3" mortars. Most were stolen over the years from the British army or purchased in the open market and then concealed in well-designed hiding places in several locations around the country. Ammunition was in short supply -- we had to report what's left following every action.

I was sent for a one-week secret assignment to kibbutz Hulata. I was led there to the farm's chicken coops area and met with my two teammates for the week.

One empty chicken coop structure was reserved for us, divided by jute partitions into three rooms. The first room contained a tall pile of round metal land mines recently pulled out of a secret hiding. Our job was to pry the mines open and collect the TNT explosive powder into the middle room. It took us a week to complete the job, ending up with a pile some 6 feet high of pure TNT. We slept in the third room and ate at the kibbutz's dining hall. The entire project was concealed from most kibbutz members.

Returning to Daphna, our squad of ten began extensive training both in field maneuvers and use of various weapons. We were old friends from Tel-Aviv, some from as far back as kindergarten. My personal weapon was a Bren light machine gun, and I treated it as if my life were dependent on it. I kept it "tuned" and under my bed at night. I was skilled at firing very short bursts, consistent with the policy of saving ammo. But often during action, when on the ground and using the bi-pod, I switched to a single-shot mode and used it like a sniper rifle. Most any target within two to three hundred yards was a sure hit. I prided myself with the growing score that I kept, never thinking of the human consequences on the other side. I just turned eighteen, was armed with a light machine gun, and given a license to shoot and kill. It gave me an intoxicating sense of power and invincibility.

In the early stages of the war, before going into action, our platoon commander would select the best "fighters" from the entire group rather than utilizing structured squads. The possibility of not being selected always raised severe anxiety in me; I could not bear the thought of not being considered a top "fighter."

We began to see more action on a regular basis. Once we rushed to extricate a bus stuck on the road by an Arab village; we had to gain control over the area before extricating the bus. On another occasion we had intelligence of a known terrorist crossing the border from Lebanon and spending the night at a specific house in an Arab village. We snuck our way at night into the village, caught the terrorist in bed, and eliminated him. We made sure to spare the life of the woman he was with.

The roads in the Galilee traversed both Arab and Jewish villages and towns. Our vehicles were subject to attacks, and we switched to convoys guarded by armored vehicles. Often, we would have to fight our way through Arab areas. This was unsustainable, consuming too many resources that we were short of. It was clear we had to strive to create a contiguous Jewish safe territory.

The most significant war action I experienced took place on 12 January 1948. Our squad of 10 had spent the prior night marching to another kibbutz about 6 miles away to bring back weapons from their secret hiding place. We each carried back three rifles or other material, returning home at about 3:00 a.m. thoroughly wet from the rain and river crossings. After breakfast our squad was called for action; the Arabs had blocked a road with rocks about a mile away and we were charged with clearing it. Our squad mounted a pickup truck and off we went. I was wearing sandals because my shoes and socks were still all wet. We thought we'd simply clear the roadblock and come straight back home. As we got close to the roadblock, we were subjected to heavy fire from two sides. We jumped off the pickup and took cover. My legs sank into the wet mud and I lost the sandals. For the next six hours I was running barefoot in the fields carrying and using the Bren gun.

We were fortunate to be led by an outstanding squad leader who managed the battle brilliantly. Throughout the battle, he issued commands as if he were moving chess pieces on the board.

We first managed to clear the roadblock and then surprised the Arabs by fighting our way forward towards another kibbutz, named K'far Szold, rather than backward -- into the waiting ambush. It took us some six hours of movement and open field fighting to reach the outskirt of our target kibbutz. By then it was about 3:00 p.m. I was crossing a plowed field leading to the gate when I fell to the ground in the middle with cramps in both legs. I was totally immobile while bullets were hitting the ground around me. Our commander came to check on me and fell by me with a bullet in his belly; yet, he continued to lead the battle. Another warrior arrived and began to operate my Bren gun, but he too was hit in a matter of minutes. We were saved by the early shadow of the winter day that covered our area. A crew with a stretcher came out of the kibbutz to bring us in. Later on, it was reported the Arabs sustained between 30 to 40 casualties.

This action was recognized after the war by being included on the list of the most exemplary and successful actions of the 1948 War of Independence, with our commander, Israel Dror, receiving a special recognition. Receiving such recognition was most uncommon in those days.

Being a small country, the word must have gotten around. In the next letter I received from my father he innocently asked, "And what happened to your sandals?" More importantly, he informed me of his latest contribution to the cause, stating: "I wanted you to know that I successfully avoided paying the due income tax to the 'soon to depart' British authorities and instead sent the money to the Jewish Agency, the Israeli government in waiting." My father's action was consistent with the spirit of the time, and I was so proud of him.

For years I have been amazed at myself at how cool and functional I was throughout the battle, until some fifty years later, with no apparent trigger, I found myself at home one evening shaking and sweating with memory of bullets whistling and buzzing by. That's part of the price we pay later on in life.

Several weeks after this battle I was ordered, along with five other members of our Daphna group, to go to the next Palmach squad command-training course. It was wartime, and I did it enthusiastically.

The training course was held in kibbutz Dalia, located some 10 miles east of Haifa in an isolated mountain area. The campsite at the kibbutz has been used for years by the Palmach underground for training its command corp. We stayed in large tents, each with some six beds. This was the first training course where all participants have already had battle experience. The war was raging throughout the country and there was a need for rapidly expanding the command ranks. Conditions in the cold and rainy winter were almost primitive, but that never bothered us. I felt honored and privileged to be a part of this elite group.

The course consisted of six weeks of intensive military training. Upon graduation, we all knew we were going back to a raging war. Newspapers carried long lists of fallen soldiers on a daily basis. Living in a small country, names were often familiar to me. As we shook hands and hugged at departure time, I kept wondering how many I might never see again.

The six of us returned to the Galilee in the early part of April 1948 and discovered our entire Daphna group had been relocated from kibbutz Daphna to the historic Tel Hai settlement. We lived in the same quarters occupied in 1920 by Yoseph Trumpeldor and his heroic comrades who lost their lives defending the place from Arab attackers. I felt deeply inspired and proud living in an actual national monument for heroes.

No more farming; this was war, and the Palmach command had taken full charge. I was glad to find my personal effects, including the violin, well in place in Tel Hai. Our new platoon commander was "Dudu" (David Tcherkasky) who went on to become a heroic mythological figure after the war.

I was in top physical condition, filled with self-confidence, and ready for my next assignment.

About one week after arrival, the six of us took part in a day-long operation in our own neighborhood. A supply convoy was being attacked south of the Arab town called Halsa (today Kiriat Sh'mone). To help in extricating it, we were attached to a force that gained control over Halsa to relieve the pressure on the convoy. I was amazed at myself how cool I was during the entire operation, when bullets were buzzing in the air close by, "zoom" and "whoof."

The big day for me came on the morning of 19 April. I was given command of a squad made up of young new recruits. Our assignment was to man a small two-story stone structure called Jahula along the main south/north road in the Hula Valley. We were to secure the road and keep an eye over the Jewish agricultural fields in the area. We arrived in early afternoon, replacing another squad that had been there for some time. The road ran along the valley's western foothills and the Nebbi Yusha fortress was immediately west of us, atop the 2,000 ft. mountain ridge. The British built it during World War II, and most recently they turned it over to the Arabs, awarding them a superior strategic advantage over all of Northern Galilee.

Nebbi Yusha Battle

In late afternoon of the same day I noticed unusual traffic of our troops on the road going south; it was obvious that something big was in the wind. The troubling thought of being stuck in this lonely outpost while the boys were going to see real action was nagging at me.

Resolution came before dark when a pick-up truck arrived with orders for us to join the assembly area in kibbutz Hulata; there was going to be an operation to capture the Nebbi Yusha fortress. I breathed a sigh of relief, and off we went.

In Hulata, I was directed to join the meeting of all in command to hear the battle plans and assignments. In the center of the large room was a large sand box depicting the grounds around the fortress, with the fortress on top carved out of a big cube of laundry soap. Moshe K., the area commander, described the plan and assignments.

The plan consisted of feigning a major attack from the south side to draw the defenders' attention, while the attacking force was sneaking up from the north, quietly cutting its way through the barbed-wire fences and setting explosives against the fortress' wall to pierce a big opening, then charging into the building to defeat the enemy. Deception, surprise, and cover of night were key elements of the plan.

Of the several questions raised following the commander's battle plan presentation, one in particular has remained stuck in my memory; it was asked by Seffie, who was a seasoned squad leader: "What happens if the Hamduni tribe that inhabited the plains immediately to the north of the fortress decided to interfere and attack us from the north?" to which Moshe, the commander, responded: "This will not happen!" In future years, this troubling exchange has repeated itself in my nightmares.

Being the lowest on the command totem pole, I didn't have the nerve to raise questions, but deep in my heart I felt the plan was very risky. Our training and actions thus far had only been at the squad and platoon levels at most, and here for the first time we had a company-level operation of eighty strong that required Swiss-watch-like precision. In addition, every single phase of it had to succeed to make it whole, and that was a bit too much to expect.

Dudu, our platoon commander, was given charge of the northern attacking force. A significant part of the force consisted of members of our Daphna group, including my four remaining friends from our recent Palmach command-training course.

My squad of riflemen was assigned to the field operation commander, Itzik, providing security to the command post that would be established on the south side. While I was proud of having my first command, I felt my assignment was of a far lesser risk and consequence than those given to my comrades and brothers in the north side. It haunts me to this day.

A company under Philon's command was charged with feigning an attack from the south/east side of the fortress. The company consisted of recently arrived young Holocaust survivors, some still barely speaking Hebrew. They loved their young leader and treated him like a young father, following him to the ends of the earth.

Two heavy machine guns were positioned directly to the south to provide fire cover for Philon's unit. The command post was placed some 50 yards behind the machine guns. I positioned my squad immediately to the left side (west) of the machine guns, about 200 yards from the fortress.

Two-way radio communication was used for coordination between the north and south forces.

Zero hour was set for midnight, providing us with some three and a half hours of remaining total night cover. According to intelligence, there were two barbed-wire fences that needed to be breached. The force also carried a long tube with explosives to be used in case breaching the fence with hand tools presented an impossible task. That was a grave planning oversight -- the use of explosives to blow up a fence would alert the defenders and the element of surprise would be lost.

Our total force of 80 left Hulata on trucks. The southern force was let off first and began its climb up the 2,000 ft. ridge, followed by the northern force, one half mile or so up the road.

From the outset we encountered logistic problems. Mainly, the trucks arrived late, and scaling the 2,000 ft. ridge took longer than expected. The zero hour kept slipping, finally settling at 3:00 a.m., 30-45 minutes before the break of dawn's light. This was the single most tragic mistake by our command, that they did not grasp the consequences of losing the cover of night.

The operation began with Philon's unit feigning the attack from the south side while the machine guns were spraying the fortress' tower with heavy fire. The northern force began cutting the barbed-wire fences.

After cutting through two fences, the northern force discovered an unexpected third one. With early dawn light approaching, they decided to explode the tube under it and rush to the wall. I remember hearing the explosion and momentarily thinking the wall had been breached. Unfortunately, with the explosion the force lost the element of surprise. The defenders began dropping hand grenades from well-protected positions above, making it impossible for anyone to reach the wall. Dudu and his crew were killed in a heroic attempt to reach the wall and set off the explosives.

The early-morning eastern sky was dawning, and with that, we lost our cover of darkness. We were caught in a barren area, exposed to enemy fire.

A retreat order was given. The machine guns on the south side were being disassembled while my squad was providing fire cover, shooting at firing positions in the fortress' tower. It was at that stage that I was hit by a bullet to the left side of the skull. I thought I was dying, but actually I fell into a coma that lasted some eight days.

The retreat of the northern force was most costly and difficult; they were caught on the barren mountain slope, taking fire from both the fortress above and the

Hamduni tribesmen on the plains north of the fortress. Several warriors from our Daphna group, following our ethos of not leaving a brother behind, tried desperately to rescue their wounded comrades and ended losing their own lives. The number of heroic acts were too many to count. Altogether we lost twelve beautiful young men from our Daphna group; some were my childhood friends. Altogether the northern force suffered nineteen casualties.

The company feigning an attack from the south lost its commander, Philon, and two soldiers. While the unit was retreating, Philon stayed behind with two seriously wounded soldiers. Recognizing he could not rescue them, and that the Arabs mutilated the wounded and did not take prisoners, he chose to end their lives with pistol shots and then shot himself.

In future years, Philon's action has given birth to discussions in Israeli military circles under the title "The Commander's Dilemma."

Altogether a total of twenty-two young men were lost in this battle, including Kuty and Yelly, from our recent Palmach command-training course. Of the original six in the course, in a matter of about one month, two were killed and two wounded. This was the war.

The pain of losing so many of our close-knit members, particularly in a losing operation, was more than unbearable. It deeply affected every member of our Daphna group and bonded us under a dark cloud hovering over us for the rest of our lives. The rage and shame over the defeat had been locked inside me for many decades, compounded by my reluctance to say anything that might appear to sully the Palmach's reputation.

One month after our failed operation, another Palmach unit captured the fortress with a loss of two soldiers. Learning from our mistakes, they first gained control over the surrounding area and then put the fortress under siege. The Arab defenders abandoned the fortress at night and escaped with their lives.

Many of our Daphna brothers' decaying bodies were found in the field in pairs--the wounded one and his rescuer. All the bodies were buried in a common grave by the fortress, which has become a national monument honoring the heroes who won't leave a brother behind.

Our Daphna Palmach unit continued to fight in the Northern front. Later on, it took part in both the Central region and Negev campaigns. All told, we suffered sixteen casualties during the war.

Following the war, members of the Daphna group formed a new kibbutz, named Yiron, located on the Lebanese border some ten miles west of the Nebbi

Yisha fortress. It is now noted for its fine winery and several manufacturing enterprises.

A good number continued with higher education and achieved successful careers in science, engineering, education, and medicine. Several members have achieved high-level positions in government and industry. One member has served a term in the Israeli Kneset.

Ten men of the Daphna group have ultimately left the country, eight to the USA and two to Europe. It's significant to note that nine out of the ten took part in the tragic Nebbi Yusha battle. Clearly, one way or another, the battle has left its deep mark on all of us.

The Rescue

During the year following the attack, I was gradually able to gather some information to reconstruct what happened to me. It was not always easy, because friends were reluctant to talk. The shame of defeat and pain of losing so many friends was unbearable. I myself was reluctant to dig in too deeply, being afraid of discovering things I would not wish to hear.

It was only forty years later that I gained the confidence and desire to pursue information in full detail.

My squad of fresh recruits was at a loss, seeing their commander "dead" on the ground with an open head wound. They were left leaderless in the field of fire. Luckily, Aharon, my friend since kindergarten who was part of the machine-gun crew, passed by and saw me. He reached the command post and reported this to Itzik, the operation commander. The two returned to the field of fire and together with two of my soldiers carried me out. The entire southern force then retreated about one mile south to the small Jewish settlement Ramot Naftali. I was placed there in a first aid station and left behind while the group proceeded to scale down the mountain and reach home base in the valley below. That was early Tuesday morning.

On Wednesday night, a unit of our Daphna group unit scaled the 2,000 ft. ridge again, carrying critical supplies for Ramot Naftali, which at the time was under siege. On their way back, they had planned to evacuate the nine infants under age two who were living there. They also had a doctor with them. To their surprise, they found me still alive, which raised a debate. Many did not think they could successfully carry me at night down the steep slope of the rough canyon while keeping the stretcher horizontal. The option of mercy killing was discussed, but the doctor insisted on giving the rescue a try.

I was tied down to a stretcher, and eight brothers carried me down the mountain. From time to time they stopped for a break, exchanging roles with those carrying the babies. Once they reached the valley, a vehicle took us to kibbutz Ayelet Hashachar, and I was placed in the medical clinic.

A medic was checking me and failed to detect a pulse; assuming I had expired, he covered my head. This was observed by Tiva, a dear high school friend who was serving in the Palmach. As she wrote in her book, she rushed to check me again and was able to detect a faint pulse, immediately calling for the doctor's help. This was now over 48 hours since injury.

Tamar was one of the kibbutz's early settlers. Her husband, Yehuda, was my father's first cousin. During my stay in the Galilee, I became close with their family, like a home away from home. I had seen Tamar about one week earlier when I was riding an armored vehicle on a mission to their kibbutz. Tamar was on duty at the medical clinic when I was brought in from Ramot Naftali and was my caregiver, and yet did not recognize me until given my name. She told me this story when I visited her several months later.

Special arrangements were made to fly me on a light aircraft from the Galilee in the north to the Beilinson hospital near Tel-Aviv, where a highly skilled neurosurgeon was available. I presume I arrived there late Thursday afternoon. I went into surgery Friday morning, over 72 hours after the injury.

II.
MAKING A LIFE
FOR MYSELF

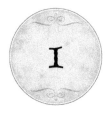

At Home

Back at home from a month in convalescence I was feeling very comfortable, stable, and safe. I was so lucky to have this home that provided me with all the support and security I needed. This was my real home, the only one I had, and I was lucky to have the freedom to pursue all my interests.

Only six weeks earlier, my reality had been war and combat, with the associated tension and sense of excitement of doing something very important, shoulder-to-shoulder with my comrades. The change was so stark, dream-like; it was like coming back from another planet, another reality. It was so peaceful and quiet at home, no pressure at all, purposeless, emptiness, and being alone and isolated. I felt like I was thrown to the sideline while real life and action were continuing out there without me.

It was now upon me alone to reconstitute my own life.

I missed my comrades and the action, the one-for-all and all-for-one spirit. I felt bad I was not shoulder-to-shoulder with them. Yet, I was secretly relieved I'd never again be faced with the paralyzing fear I experienced during the few moments before battle began, before the first shot was fired. It was a conflict I could not resolve; both feelings were within me.

Health-wise, I had managed to gain some weight and increase my energy level. My right hand was "useless" – it felt like I was wearing a thick boxing glove. I had no feeling in my fingers, could not discern textures, and had no sense of space or location. Without looking at my hand, I could not do anything with it; I could not tell where it was. The entire arm seemed weak and disoriented.

My speech was improving, at times a bit hesitantly. My vision was fine, but I still had some difficulty reading -- the letters jumping up and down. I was very protective of my head with a 4X4" hole under the skin over the left ear; I was feeling vulnerable and cautious.

I was very sensitive to direct sun and hot summer days. Just as critical were the effects of being on Luminal as a precaution against seizure; in later years it was changed to Dilantin. It had a slowing-down effect and it forced me to maintain a well-structured life, like having a regular 8 hours of sleep every night. If I missed one night, my effectiveness the next day would sharply suffer.

I was confident that with time I could overcome most of my difficulties, if not all, and learn to finesse around them if necessary. I also knew my life had taken a big turn and I needed to work on making adjustments. I had to protect my skull, and that meant a change in a way of life; there were situations I needed to avoid.

I did not consider myself disabled, but only saddled with some restrictions that were a part of life. I must adjust to the new me, my new reality, my new normal.

I did not internalize the amazing miracle of my medical recovery and did not give it much thought. In my mind it was like "I was shot in the head, thought I was dying, woke up in a hospital, now I am among the living and my task now is to physically heal and get better." I was in total denial and afraid to touch the areas of emotional pain and feelings. I never mourned the loss of my physical capabilities; rather, attacking the problems became my way of being. I was consumed with the notion that I must do the best with what I had and continue to improve myself.

The war was raging on, and I was home safe. It was both a pleasant and disturbing feeling; at times I felt like I was a deserter. It was very personal; it was my war, my friends' and my generation's. Yet, I was sitting safely on the sideline and my good brothers were out there fighting and risking their lives. These conflicting feelings were eating me up inside.

Friends visited me during the war's lull periods. Ely, my high school seatmate for four years, came to see me. He was in a different unit and we had not seen each other since graduation some ten months earlier. He was an exceptional fine, solid, straight-arrow, talented young man. One week after the visit, he was killed in action—he took a bullet to his forehead. The pain I hide is with me forever, added to the long list of hurts I harbor. I kept it all in because life goes on and "this is what strong men do."

At home, there was never a conversation with my parents about feelings, mine or theirs, of having experienced their young son's life almost being lost. I remember only one comment my mother once made to me during the entire year: "For us, it's as if you were born all over again, like a new son."

Once I was well enough to walk around, my father asked that I visit his company's office to greet his many colleagues. It was his way of showing his pride in both my war exploits and miraculous recovery. I was amazed at the extra-warm reception I received; I did not see myself as exceptional. The office manager, a true old-timer wearing a big thick mustache, came to hug me; as was customary at the time, he also knelt down to kiss the ground I was standing on. He was really honoring all the Palmach soldiers, the spearhead of the new Israeli army, who were shouldering the war's heaviest burden. The memory of the event has stayed with me forever.

The Moskowitz family lived two blocks away from us; their son Mal'achy was one of the twelve killed from our Daphna group. Mal'achy and I were in the same high school class. Our respective fathers were business acquaintances. At first opportunity, I paid my respects with a condolence visit. They were devastated; Sonia, his mother, took to wearing only black garments; Baruch, his father, remained stoic and was very bitter. I was speechless and did not know what to say. I thought just being there would deliver the message that I cared and had not forgotten their son. I found myself duty-bound to visit them on a regular basis. Every visit was the same -- we were just sitting there, saying little, me listening to their painful talk.

On a stroll in our neighborhood I was surprised to run into Menachem Shuval, a member of our Daphna group, originally from the scout troops in Haifa. We were only casual friends then, but this was wartime and we embraced warmly. He turned to me and said: "Amnon, I'm so glad to see you alive. You won't believe me, but I was one of the guys who carried you down the mountain on a stretcher, and you were so damn heavy! I was praying you'd survive so that I'd have the opportunity to damn you in person for being so heavy! So here it is: Damn you, Amnon, you were so damned heavy!"

I was dumbfounded and taken aback. Here was one of my lifesavers, and I still knew so little about the entire story; for some reason, I was not too actively searching for it.

Catching my breath, I responded, "And I want to express my deep gratitude to you for doing all this for me," and he said, "Oh Amnon, forget it; I know you'd have done exactly the same thing for me!"

He was so right--I would have done it in a heartbeat. I also realized at that moment it was so much easier for me to give, even risking my life in battle, than to receive. How do I ever pay back for all those who saved my life? Just saying "thank you" would never be enough.

The unfulfilled feeling of my need to give back has remained with me for the rest of my life, compounded by the guilt feelings for not standing shoulder-to-shoulder in combat with my comrades for the rest of the war. At times, I felt like a deserter who somehow managed to get out of the fighting way before war's end.

We parted ways after some more small talk. Little did we know that forty years later, Menachem would play another key role in my life.

On the first year's battle anniversary, three days before the Passover holiday, a major memorial was held at the common gravesite by the Nebbi Yusha fortress. Sitting next to me on the special bus from Tel-Aviv was Robert Abraham Bartfeld, a high school classmate and a member of our Daphna group. Bob was a member of the unit attacking the fortress from the north side. It was our first meeting since the battle, and we exchanged our stories.

I told Bob about my actions, from the south side, shortly before being shot, that I was shooting directly at the firing holes in the tower on top of the fortress, adding that I thought I was scoring some hits.

Bob's response was amazing, claiming I actually may have saved his life! He proceeded to tell me that during the retreat, he kept jumping between hiding places, evading enemy fire coming from the tower. At one point, the fire remained focused on him and he was trapped behind a rock for some time. Suddenly the firing from the tower stopped. and he was able to extricate himself. He put two and two together and decided it was my shots at the tower that saved his life. Of course, there was no way on earth to truly link between the two events, but Bob chose to adopt the belief that I was responsible for saving his life.

Bob and I had an unbreakable lifelong bond, although we did not see one another often. He spent his entire career as a professor of engineering in Wisconsin. Late in life, he suffered from kidney failure and went on dialysis. When he finally decided to terminate the treatment, he called me to bid farewell, passing on two days later. Bob was a gentle hero.

During the entire memorial ceremony, I felt numb, distant, flat, and alone. I harbored shame of survival--why me and not them? But I was unable to express anything. I felt I got away easy. I survived; my task was relatively "safe," while my dead brothers took the heavy risk and paid the ultimate price. They were the heroes while I underperformed; I failed their trust. Underneath there was also a great deal of rage, which I was unable to clearly identify or express. I wanted to get away. For almost twenty years I did not visit Nebbi Yusha again.

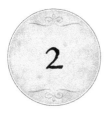

Physical Rehab At Home

While at the convalescent home, I was just "existing." I was very tired, and I needed to rest myself both physically and mentally. I needed time to sort things out. I was just happy to be, my mind shut off from the rest of the world. It seemed like I was in some sort of a daze.

Upon returning home from convalescence, I began to assess my situation. I was faced with the fact that I literally lost the use of my right hand, my dominant hand. If I were to re-enter mainstream life and regain the ability to actualize myself in the world, to pursue my ambitions to the fullest, I needed to rehabilitate the use of my right hand. I did not want to lead the life of a disabled person but was willing to accept some limitations and do the best I could with what I had. Bringing my right hand to at least a useful level was foremost on my mind.

When I was released from the hospital I was given no medical, rehab, or psychological advice; it was more like "Your life has been saved; now you are on your own." My doctors told me the future of my right hand was "in the hands of the Creator," but I believed I must do something about it -- take control.

Regaining my physical conditioning was paramount, so I began with what I knew -- calisthenics. We used to do them at school every morning before classes, so I was back to the same routine, every morning for about 20 minutes. I also added pushups for good measure. Within a few months, my physical conditioning was back to normal. It was an exercise routine I continued for decades to come.

My right hand was a much greater challenge. I first did the easy thing -- muscular development. I got a spring-loaded device for exercising the grip and I used it often throughout the day. The hand muscles were coming back to life.

As I was doing the calisthenics, I wanted to make sure the "weak" right arm was participating fully, so I moved to the hallway in front of a large mirror. With eyes open I could ensure that both arms were doing the same thing -- a mirror image of each other. I then realized that in forcing the right arm and hand to mirror the left I was creating new habits, new control, or new brain paths.

With the new insight, I added making freestyle symmetrical movements with both my arms and hands in front of the mirror; it was like a dance, or breast strokes in the water: whatever I did must be symmetrical. The right side was learning from the healthy left, being guided with my eyes. I was creating new paths in the brain.

Freestyle symmetrical movements with my arms in front of the mirror was something I was doing repeatedly every day, again, again and again. Now I was like a free-form dancer in front of the mirror and having fun doing it.

I accomplished muscular control of my right arm and hand, but the "feeling" function of the fingers was gone forever. The control is based in the brain and the damage was permanent.

The use of table utensils with my right hand was target number one. I was determined not to become "left-handed" by default. I treated the right hand as an uneducated limb that needed to be taught how to function, like a computer without a program.

I began by placing the right hand on the table, palm up. That took some doing; I actually used the left hand to place the right palm in place. With my left hand, I placed a fork on the palm and wrapped the fingers around it. I made sure I had a secure grip. Next, I lifted the right arm and made motions simulating the feeding process, from the plate to the mouth. I would repeat this over and over, creating "new paths," creating a routine. I had a lot of patience and all the time in the world.

I discovered the most difficult part of this process was the initial grabbing of the fork. Once it was in my hand, I found that with training and time I made really good progress. So I decided to adapt and not to fight the impossible. I reached for the fork with my left and transferred it to the right. It worked. Still, it took practice, practice, and practice to make it happen. Years later, I became more advanced by learning to pick up the fork with my right hand; it's not perfect, but it works.

I remember one morning at breakfast I was sitting at the kitchen table eating scrambled eggs prepared by my mother. She was sitting across the table watching with great pleasure every move I made. Suddenly my right hand missed the target -- the fork with scrambled egg struck my right cheek instead of the mouth. She became a bit teary, and I had to assure her that things would improve; it's only the beginning, not to worry.

This rehab thing was not a one-time effort, it has become my way of life. It has never stopped. I continually test myself how far I can go. Even now, over seventy years later, I challenge myself every time I pick up the fork -- can I do it without the assistance of my left hand? It's a way of life, and it's also a game.

The same was true when it came to writing. I refused to become a "lefty." The process was similar to the one I used for table utensils. I first spread a large sheet of paper on a table, then I grabbed the right palm with my left hand and placed it on the table, palm up. With my left hand, I placed a pencil in the palm, then closed the fingers on it using my left hand, creating a grip. Now my left hand grabbed the right fist and turned it over. Using the arm's muscles, I began to draw freehand lines. After a while, I began to draw straight lines, vertical and horizontal. I finally dared to draw a large square and a large circle. After some practice, I began to draw smaller squares and circles. I kept repeating this every day over and over, and after a while I began to draw large letters and numbers, several inches high. As confidence grew, I was drawing smaller and smaller letters. It all took time, of which I was fortunate to have plenty.

After a great deal of practice, I took a stab at writing my first letter, a short one and using block letters, addressed to my older brother Yehuda who was studying at U. C. Berkeley. That was my victory dance! Over a period of time I was able to write in script, although my handwriting was not the same as before, but who cared?

Repetition and patience were the hallmarks of success in this game. I was stubborn and confident I could make it. I was also not embarrassed or ashamed at not being as good as before. On the contrary, I was proud of my achievements. I was doing the best I could with what I had.

The only way I can securely do anything with the right hand is by watching every move with my eyes. After a lot of practice, I was developing a new eye-hand connection. Playing the violin was absolutely impossible; I could not hold the bow, let alone have subtlety of control over the strings. I started studying violin at age six, and music has been an important part of my life. I have easily mastered playing other instruments as well, like mandolin, trumpet, recorder, and harmonica. My mother was very musical and had a fine singing voice. I grew up listening to her singing while she was doing her housework in the mornings; I can still sing the tunes I learned from her.

I decided to turn adversity to advantage: "If I could not play the violin, why not play the accordion? It's a win-win for me." I could enjoy the music while exercising the right-hand fingers on the keyboard! Exercise was what I needed most!

From idea to action, I bought an accordion and took lessons for about three months, principally learning the instrument and the chord system controlled by the left hand. Another challenge I was facing was playing while looking at the music score; I could either look at the score or at my right hand, not both. I must constantly watch the right-hand fingers to guide them on the keyboard. I solved this by memorizing the score, fortunately an easy task for me.

The last issue I had to address was my own brain function. The fact that I suffered a brain injury created doubts within me that perhaps I may have lost some of my native capacity. Mathematics and science were my strong subjects at school and I felt I needed to test and exercise my brain. I turned to the game of chess.

I practically grew up at home with the game of chess; it was my father's main recreation. Friday afternoon was a chess-playing party at home with his small group of friends, and Saturday morning they played at a friend's house two doors down the street. They were expert players that took the game very seriously. It seemed like I learned the game by osmosis when a very young boy, but I never invested much time actually playing it.

Being alone, my approach was analyzing tournament games played by the great international Grand Masters. I purchased M. Botvinik's book in which he annotated each of the sixty games played in the 1941 contest for the USSR chess championship, which he won on his way to winning the world championship.

At times, I could easily spend two to three hours a day studying the masters' games. It took a lot of concentration and brainwork. Later on, I used other tournament books written by other chess grand masters.

Rehabbing my right hand has become a way of life for me; it never stopped. I made most gains in the first three to six months, but the challenge has never stopped, even as I was writing this page. I must think every time I use the right hand, so the battle memories are awakened every moment of my life. Life's minutiae take me longer to do -- buttoning my shirt, tying shoelaces -- and I need to factor that time into my daily routines. I have integrated it into my daily routines and it has become my new normal. It's not a handicap; it's a normal.

My condition also called for creative problem-solving. For instance, the only object I keep in my right trousers pocket is my key chain. Because of its bulk and large, odd shape, I can "fish" it out of my pocket with my non-feeling right fingers. Whatever I manage to hook onto, it must be the key chain.

At times I surprise myself with my progress. For twenty years I was happily playing the accordion, never giving a thought to the violin. One of my colleagues at work was an advanced amateur pianist who kept encouraging me to give the violin a try while I kept dismissing it. One day he gave me a newspaper clipping with an ad -- someone was selling a violin for $100. I didn't know what got into me, but I followed up and bought the instrument; not much to lose, another "toy." Yet, much to my surprise I was taken by the challenge. I discovered I could manage to hold the bow with my right hand, not exactly in the classic way, but good enough to produce good sound. So, I got into it seriously. I began to practice every evening, starting with the very basics, like drawing the bow over the open strings. I proceeded with playing scales and gaining skill and confidence. After about one year I was playing some of the mid-level concertos that I had played in my youth.

Then came another surprise. Another colleague at work told me his wife was playing with a local community orchestra. "Why don't you join?" -- which I did. I was seated at the last chair of the Second Violin section. We rehearsed every Monday evening and performed in concert several times a year. One thing I absolutely could not do was play pizzicato while holding the bow with my hand, so I was faking it, letting the audience think I was actually doing it. The conductor was aware of my condition and played along.

Playing the violin has become an important part of my life, and I continue to enjoy it immensely. Later in life I was fortunate to acquire a fine handmade instrument with a wonderful voice; playing it gives me indescribable emotional pleasure. Because of my right hand, I am technically limited with what I can play, but all I want is the enjoyment of making the beautiful sound of music.

I must highlight another example of "long-term rehab." I once bought a new car and drove it for twelve years. The starter keyhole was mounted on the right side of the steering column, which meant I had to hold the key with my right hand and carefully search for the keyhole. I developed the habit of leaning to the right until I could visually see the keyhole, then carefully inserting the key to start the car.

I don't know when, but some years into ownership I discovered that even with my eyes closed, I could swing my arm with the key and insert it precisely into the keyhole. The only requirement was that I first made sure my hand was holding the key at the correct angle. Clearly, the shoulder muscles have learned the routine through repetition. This was strictly a case of muscle memory; good enough for me.

Regardless of the great progress I have made in rehabilitating my right hand and fingers, the biggest impact on my life has remained the battle reminder that stays alive with me every moment of my life, particularly when I use my right hand. It's a subliminal message that at times seems to fade away but always comes back. It is a part of who I have become.

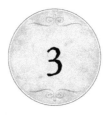

Dr. Askenasy

Professor Dr. Harden Askenasy received his advanced medical training in the USA and Canada before returning to his native Romania in the late 1930s to become chief of neurosurgery at Bucharest's central hospital. Having survived the Holocaust, he and his wife managed to get on a refugee boat heading towards the Promised Land but ended up being detained by the British in a Cyprus camp. They finally arrived in Israel in late March or early April 1948, when The War of Independence was raging on. I owe my life to Dr. Askenasy, and so do hundreds of other soldiers and civilians.

From time to time during my rehab year I would visit Dr. Askenasy at his Tel-Aviv clinic. I was receiving the VIP treatment and would be let in without waiting in line. My need to see him was emotional; there was nothing medical he could do for me any more. I gained confidence from the satisfied and self-assured expression in his eyes. He brought me back to life, and I could see his delight in seeing me doing so well. I considered him to be a second father.

On several occasions he invited me to medical lectures where I was shown as a medical case study. I was more than happy to comply -- I had such great confidence in him I'd follow his advice to the edge of the earth. I would be presented to the audience and asked to perform arm movements with my eyes shut, such as touching my nose with the index finger.

Living with a 4"X4" hole in the skull was very worrisome to me, to say the least. My brain was covered only by skin and hair. Any sharp blow to the area would be fatal. I had to be extra careful whenever I moved. I shared my concerns with Dr. Askenasy. His answer was very clear. "Amnon, if you wished, I could install a plate now, but I do not recommend it. You are young, and your skull continues to change shape. If I installed a plate now, I can assure you it'd give you trouble soon, and we'd have to remove it. If you can handle it, I recommend you wait a few years." I did not think twice; I took his advice to heart and deferred the issue for a few years. It meant I had to adjust my lifestyle, such as avoiding crowded and unruly situations.

Dr. Askenasy was also responsible for my decision to go abroad for my academic studies. The option of studying at the Haifa Technion was very attractive--a great school and close to home. That was the mood at home with my protective parents. My older brother, Yehuda, was studying at the time at U.C. Berkeley in California, one of the top public universities in the USA.

My father and I went to see Dr. Askenasy to get his opinion on this matter. I will never forget his response. "Let him go," he said to my father, while waving his arm away from his body. "Let him go; he needs to get away." He saw something in me that I was totally unaware of and I am sure my parents could not see either--the post-traumatic stress effects on me. He knew I needed to get away, to get some distance from my current reality. For this, again, I will forever be grateful to my doctor, this great human being.

So the decision was made. When ready, I would go to school at U.C. Berkeley in California.

Me and the VA

After several months at home, my case was transferred from the military to the Disabled Veterans Affairs under the Defense Department. I met with my case officer, Olga S., to get acquainted and discuss the future. I was issued new documents and discovered I was awarded 65% disabilities.

After several meetings we got to the subject of "the future." The system was very kind to me; they wanted to be sure I could earn a decent living despite my disabilities. It was a bit strange to me: I didn't see myself as disabled, only as "limited" in certain areas. I saw myself as a healthy person, striving to become even healthier. At that time, the emotional component was the farthest thing from my mind. I was in a total and absolute state of denial.

Two attractive options were being offered to me to choose from: a 50% partnership in a movie theater or a "green number," meaning a taxi cab license which I could lease to others. Either one could earn me nice income.

I turned both offers down and asked instead that they give me a stipend to a university. This must have been a surprise to them, particularly coming from a young soldier with a serious head injury. I was asked to undergo a psychological evaluation and issued an appointment with a psychiatrist.

I showed up for the appointment; it turned out the office was adjacent to Dr. Askenasy's clinic. The psychiatrist was seated behind a big heavy desk and I was asked to sit in front of him as I watched him browsing through my medical file. After a while he began asking me questions. He pointed to an ashtray on the desk and asked, "Amnon, can you tell me what this object is?"

After getting over my shock I said, "Ashtray, of course."

He then picked up a fountain pen and asked, "Amnon, and what is this object?"

Now my eyes were getting red with anger -- what did he think I was, a vegetable? I managed to contain my anger and said, "A fountain pen." In my mind I was thinking, *My God, we used to slug people for a lesser affront.*

He then picked up the little hammer they use for checking joint reflexes and asked: "Amnon, can you tell me what this is?" This was it! I had reached my limit. I looked him straight in the eyes and calmly said: "I believe this is a horse and buggy."

Now he was taken aback and becoming very agitated, realizing I was putting him on. Just at that moment there was a knock on the door and Dr. Askenasy walked in, apparently wishing to say hello to me. The psychiatrist turned to him, saying something like, "What kind of a brazen young man is Amnon? Rather disrespectful," and Dr. Askenasy replied something like, "It's OK, it's permissible; he's earned it."

The bottom line was positive for me. I was awarded a 50% stipend plus travel costs to the University of California in Berkeley. A student annual budget at the time was $1,200, so I received $600 a year plus travel. I was lucky my parents could handle the balance, and I was also able to augment the budget with some part-time work.

Berkeley, California

Arriving in Berkeley in the autumn of 1949 felt like landing on a different planet. I loved it from the first moment--the relaxed and peaceful environment, the quiet, the cleanliness, being treated with respect, and the great climate. It was heaven for me, away from the summer heat and tumult back home, but most importantly, away from the daily reminders of war and the Nebbi Yusha battle. I could let myself breathe and smile at will. I could be myself and begin a new chapter of life.

I moved in with my brother Yehuda, who was entering his senior year, which made my adjustment so much easier.

School was not a great challenge, and I also did not feel a need to ace every course I took; rather, maintaining a steady pace and staying in balance was more important to me. Still feeling a bit fragile, I needed stability; I was re-entering life again and was happy to take my time. My major was an amorphous "engineering," simply because I was strong in science, but had nothing to do with a specific career objective. After one year I realized I was just as much interested in the human side of life and I switched my major to "Industrial Management," combining the engineering subjects with business, economics and management.

Social life for Jewish students was centered around the Hillel House off campus and I was glad to provide the music playing the accordion; Israeli folk dances, polkas, and waltzes were my specialty. That's where I first saw Selma Lee Sarnoff, who was leading the folk dancing. It was love at first sight for me and we got married in the summer of 1951, before our senior year. Lee was pursuing a teaching career.

We both graduated with bachelor degrees in 1952 and moved to Los Angeles. Under my student visa, I was allowed to obtain work experience in my field for two years, while Lee needed to do one year as a student teacher before being certified.

During the two years, I was fortunate to hold two jobs that provided me with great experience. In the first one, I managed production control for an electronic parts supply and manufacturing company. In the second one, I was the industrial engineer for a small

TV-set manufacturer. In both cases, I acquired valuable experience that served me well later in my career.

After Lee completed the student-teaching year, she worked for a full year as an elementary school teacher. Together we managed to save some $5,000, which we used to purchase electrical appliances for our move to Israel.

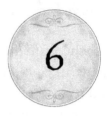

Moving to Israel

Our plan was to establish a home in Israel and start raising a family.

The first stop on our way to Israel was Detroit, visiting with my cousin Eugene. During the 1948 War of Independence, Eugene arrived in Israel as a volunteer young doctor and stayed with us for the duration. He also managed to woo and marry Anita, our next-door neighbor.

It was during the Friday evening dinner that he casually asked me, "Amnon, how was the plate in your head doing"? He assumed I had it installed before coming to the US. He was more than surprised to learn I was still without a plate, six years post injury. His reaction was swift. Without wasting a minute, he got on the phone to his colleague, Dr. Richard C. Schneider, a highly regarded neurosurgeon at the University of

Michigan in Ann Arbor. Dr. Schneider has served in WWII and was up to date on the latest neurosurgical technologies.

Saturday morning, we drove to Ann Arbor to meet with Dr. Schneider. After examining me, he stated he'd be most happy to install a plate using plastic material, which he would form to shape during surgery. The plastic material was superior to metal; it had similar material characteristics to bone and it avoided the "hot head" phenomenon associated with metal plates. My decision was a "no-brainer"--I'd go into surgery Monday morning. We drove back to Detroit the same afternoon and my cousin drove Lee and me back to Ann Arbor Sunday afternoon. Lee checked into the student dorms while I checked into the hospital.

The surgery was routine but with a big surprise. It turned out during the six years since injury, a new thin bone tissue has grown diagonally across the 4"X4" opening in the skull. The surgeon decided to leave it alone and place the plate on top of it. After two days, I was released to my cousin's care at his home in Detroit. In total the surgery caused two weeks' delay to our travel plans.

I kept counting my blessings. A courtesy visit with my cousin ended up with the best medical treatment on earth. This plate will have served me well for the rest of my life.

From Detroit we traveled to Camden, New Jersey, for a visit with Lee's family. We then traveled to New York to board a ship sailing to Le Havre, France, and on to Paris, where we picked up a car, then traveled through southern France, Northern Italy, ending up in Naples, where we, and our car, boarded the boat *Artza* for the final leg to Haifa, Israel.

Standing on the deck and watching Israel's coastline appearing over the eastern horizon evoked in me powerful emotions to the point of shedding tears of happiness. Here was the land I loved, the land I had yearned for my entire life, the land I fought for and almost lost my life for, the land so many of my good friends lost their lives for – it was right there in front of me! It was real! The mixed emotions were too powerful to contain, while I was also overcome with joy.

Both my father and brother Yehuda were waiting for us at the port. I lost it when we met and broke down crying as I was hugging my father. From an early age, as I remember, my father has been my "true north," the one person I trusted for support, kindness, ethics, and good judgment. He was suffering with a cardiac ailment but still took the arduous trip from Tel-Aviv to Haifa to greet us. It was a very happy day for him; not only was I returning home, but also bringing a bride along with whom he fell instantly in love.

Israel 1954-57

I departed Israel for Berkeley in 1949, just one year after it became an independent nation in 1948. When we returned five years later, it was in many ways like a new country for me. The rate of change during my absence was breathtaking, both in physical growth and government administration. I had to learn many things as if I were a newcomer; some of the things I liked and some less, particularly the bureaucracy. Most of all I liked the people, my family and friends, the informality, the Hebrew language, the deep historical roots, the beauty of the countryside, and the fact that it was ours.

I was concerned with some changes in attitudes that I observed. Throughout my growing years I identified myself with the pioneering idealistic Israel and by the willingness to sacrifice for the common good; my generation has lived by that rule and also paid a heavy price for it. Now I saw people were more concerned with their personal gain and advancement. Perhaps that was normal for a stable healthy society and it was me who was left behind the times, but coming back after five years, the difference was stark, and unpleasant at times.

We settled into our new cottage in a Tel-Aviv suburb and developed a full social life in our own neighborhood. It was a happy time.

I was happy to find work with the management-consulting branch of one of the country's largest CPA firms. My work got me involved with a variety of industries across the economic spectrum.

Our daughter Dana was born in November 1955, the first grandchild for my parents.

Tragedy struck only five weeks later when my father died of a heart attack at the age of fifty-one. His loss hit me very hard; he was my rock, my trusted counselor, and my ethical guidepost. I barely had a chance to develop an adult relationship with him. His early loss forced me to assume full adult responsibilities, recognizing I was on my own, all alone. My physical limitations, however invisible, made my isolation come into sharper focus.

Another turning point occurred in early in 1956 when I was called before a medical review board, although my status and disability level had already been set as "permanent." The board convened at the Hadassah hospital in Tel-Aviv. Three individuals made up the board and no medical exam took place. They examined my file, checked me visually, and I was dismissed.

Several weeks later, I received an official letter advising me my disability level was reduced from 65% to 37%. I was shocked and infuriated. This was my first significant encounter with the new bureaucracy and it was in sharp contrast to the way I was handled in 1948/9 following my injury. Now I had become a statistic at the whim of anonymous bureaucracy. This was all new to me, and I remained utterly frustrated with rage and a sense of helplessness. Old ghosts and open wounds from the Nebbi Yusha battle, buried deeply in my soul, were being raised again after five years of calm while in the USA.

In desperation I turned to my "second father," Dr. Harden Askenasy. I had already made courtesy calls on him after my return from the USA; now it was business. I told him my story and asked if there was a way he could be of help. Without hesitation, he offered to appear in front of an appeal medical board.

Again, the medical board convened at the Hadassah hospital in Tel-Aviv. Dr. Askenasy and I arrived together, but the board chose to see only him, leaving me waiting in the hallway. When he finally came out his face was ashen. He put his arm around my shoulder saying, "Amnon, let's walk away from here ... I'm sorry I could not help you. This is not a medical board; it's a political board."

I was shocked and embarrassed to have put Dr. Askenasy through this. I was upset beyond words. It became clear what the "medical" board was doing; the 50% disability level represented a big step function in benefits and the board was systematically lowering rates below the 50% level. This was not just a bureaucracy, but a corrupt one.

Later in the future I was referred once to meet with an attorney who offered to help me "fix" the problem, but I refused to follow through with the unethical path that would have made me part of the system I disliked.

I lost my encounter with the new pragmatic Israel, and I learned a bitter lesson; I felt helplessly betrayed, abandoned, and discarded. I did not have the energy to deal with these obstacles.

It was not the question of monetary compensation but an insult to the core of my being. Consistent with my rehab approach, I knew I had to become independent of this bureaucracy; I could not let them control my life. Paradoxically, this gave me greater drive to succeed in life without being dependent on government dole.

Very painfully, I realized I did not have the energy, nor skill or desire, to deal with these unpleasant challenges. I was a warrior in my youth, I have paid the price, and now my priority was seeking a productive, quiet, and uncomplicated life taking care of my family.

While my consulting work was very interesting and challenging, I was becoming increasingly aware that I was missing out on the great technological developments taking place in the USA in the fields of computing and office automation. Everything pointed in the direction of returning to the USA, both for professional development and regaining peace of mind.

I was torn between my lifelong love for and commitment to the establishment and security of the state of Israel, and my desire to lead a productive life consistent with my physical limitations and the urgent need for a peace of mind.

I kept thinking of Dr. Askenasy's hand motion and words to my father five years earlier: "Let him go." The great man knew of the turmoil in my soul long before I allowed myself to acknowledge it.

I kept thinking of Rabbi Hillel's wisdom: "If I am not for me, who will be for me? And when I am for myself alone, what am I? And if not now, then when?"

Going to the USA at that stage was a painful decision but a necessary one for both professional development and regaining peace of mind.

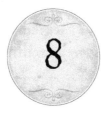

8

USA

I was trying to put everything behind me and focus on my work career and raising a family.

Our son Michael was born several months after we arrived in Los Angeles in 1957. Shortly thereafter we moved to Pittsburgh, PA, where I took a job representing a small California company selling inter-couplers for both IBM and NCR office equipment. Pittsburgh was headquarters to a large number of major US corporations, like US Steel, ALCOA, and Westinghouse, and doing business there was a valuable and exciting teaching experience. Two years later, I was promoted to our company's headquarters back in the Los Angeles area.

One year later I literally walked across the street to join the Electronics Division of NCR, becoming a member of the team designing the original online banking system; this was truly pioneering stuff in the early 1960s. I thrived in that environment. It was an ideal work situation -- I was able to both contribute and learn while doing very exciting work in a pioneering field.

As I was advancing in responsibilities, I realized I needed more training in management skills. I turned to seminars offered by The Graduate School of Business Management at UCLA, aimed at professionals in the workplace. My employer was more than happy to sponsor me. Our group of twelve individuals from different companies met once a week on campus from 4:00 to 7:00 p.m. under professional guidance. The class, or group, lasted ten weeks, or one semester. Titled "Sensitivity Training," it was group therapy for all intents and purposes.

The sensitivity training was a godsend for me. The war experience sent me into a protective shell that I dared not penetrate or talk about. I had been trying to have a career and lead a peaceful life as if the raging storm within me did not exist. In our group sessions, I began to find a safe environment where gradually, very gradually, I began to open up. It was only in the advanced group I attended the next semester that I dared to talk about my injuries and war experience. This was in contrast to my workplace environment, where I had been careful not to discuss my war injuries for fear it could affect my career progress.

UCLA was offering a variety of advanced seminars that I continued to take over several years, and I attribute my success in corporate life to the valuable lessons I learned. It also had a positive effect on our home life; several times my wife and I attended such seminars together. Yet, deep inside, the devil was still haunting me. Frequent nightmares were my utmost secrets.

In the mid-sixties I received several interesting job offers from Israeli companies. After soul-searching, I decided to continue with my promising career in the USA. The issues that were haunting me in 1957 were still in play, and there was no good reason for me to change course.

In 1966 I accepted a six-months consulting assignment with the Israel Bankers Association to conduct a feasibility study concerning computerization of the banking system in Israel. I was fortunate that my employer was willing to give me a leave of absence. It was an opportunity to expose our children to Israel and for me to hopefully make a contribution. We stayed in a rented apartment in Tel-Aviv, and the children attended local public schools. During our entire stay, I avoided visiting the Nebbi Yusha battle site; I was afraid to stir up my emotions, and I kept a protective shell around myself.

We returned to Los Angeles in the spring of 1967, a short time before the eruption of the Six Day War.

My career at NCR continued to advance and I was assigned as program manager for the design and delivery of one of the world's largest online banking systems, for the Sumitomo bank of Japan. Working closely with the Japanese and studying their culture added a new dimension to my life experience that I value highly.

First Visit to Nebbi Yusha

Israel's swift victory over its Arab neighbors in the 1967 war caused seismic changes in its geopolitics and presented enormous opportunities. I was eager to observe it first hand, so I took a quick trip back to Israel. I was able to visit both the Suez Canal and the Golan Heights.

Somehow, on a whim, I made a bold decision to visit the Nebbi Yusha fortress. It would be my first visit in eighteen years. I arrived alone at noon on a very hot day. I brought my heavy film movie camera bag, with the intention of filming the battle site from the fortress' roof.

Back in 1948 the area was totally barren; now I saw trees and shrubbery all around. Approaching the area, I felt the world had come to a standstill; it was very quiet and I knew my feet were stepping on sacred ground. I walked to the fence's gate and told the sentry I wanted to see the commanding officer. The fortress was manned by a border guard unit. When the commander arrived I said, "My name is Amnon Ben-Yehuda and I'd like to get on the roof to film the area around the fortress."

He took a long look at me, from head to toe, and after a pause said, "Come, follow me," as if he were expecting me and knew all about me. He led me to a small buffet area on the ground floor, asking, "Hot or cold?"

I said, "Cold." An orderly served us with cold drinks and we sat there resting without words. I sat there amazed at myself for being there; was it a dream?

After a while he asked, "Are you ready?"

"Yes," I said and got up.

The only way to the roof was by climbing an iron ladder that cut through the floors.

"May I carry your camera bag?" he asked, and I quietly handed him the heavy case.

I began climbing, and he was right behind me.

When we were both on the roof he handed me the case and said, "I'll leave you alone; you can stay here as long as you want," and he quietly left.

I stood there for a long time, stunned by the beauty of the 360-degree view; it was hypnotic. The Golan Heights to the east, Mt. Hermon to the north/east, and the cultivated Hula Valley fields below to the east.

I turned to the south side and easily identified the area I was at when shot. *What an easy target from here* was the thought that crossed my mind. The tragedy of our defeat filled my mind as I was crying for my lost friends.

I could not do the filming. I could not take the camera out of the case. It would be sacrilege. I was standing on sacred ground; the view was untouchable, and I was sobbing.

The commander walked me out to the gate and we said farewell. It will remain a mystery how he was able to see through me. Perhaps it was a mystery how I became so transparent on that day.

At the time I did not realize I was on a transformational path, on a long arduous path toward healing my wounded soul.

On subsequent visits in future years, I avoided entering the fortress but rather went directly to the common grave under its shadow, spending time shedding tears in solitude.

III.
THE CRISIS

In 1971, the company moved our division from the Los Angeles area to Rancho Bernardo, near San Diego. We bought a new house in San Diego and settled into our new community. It was a blessing far beyond our dreams.

Upon completion of the Sumitomo bank project, I was asked by the company to form the Special Systems Division, chartered to design and build large online systems for customers worldwide. Shortly thereafter, I was invited to join the San Diego Rotary Club, which turned out to be a major positive milestone in my life. Our family also joined a Jewish temple and we became involved in volunteer and community service activities. For the first time in the USA, I began to develop a sense of belonging and ownership in my community. All of this was most gratifying to me as a newcomer to the USA. San Diego has become my second and true hometown.

After six years of running the Special Systems Division, I accepted the challenge of running a company that NCR had acquired in Silicon Valley. We moved to that area and established a well-rounded social and cultural life.

Belatedly I discovered the acquired company was in bad financial shape and its technology was outdated. There was also an unbridgeable cultural gulf in management style between the old-fashioned Ohio-based NCR and the freewheeling Silicon Valley entrepreneurial spirit. In two years, we brought the company to a break-even point but NCR was unwilling to invest in new technologies. There was no more reason for me to continue, and we parted ways.

I began to work as an independent consultant to small hi-tech companies and was very comfortable in that role. Along the way, we moved back to San Diego, my adopted hometown, and renewed our personal connections and community activities.

I should have stuck with it, but I fell for the tempting offer to become CEO of a small software company in San Diego; running an independent company has been one of my lifelong ambitions. It was the devil in me pulling in the wrong direction at the wrong time in my life, and I made a mistake; perhaps it was the ego in me that took over. The job demanded maximum energy, and I discovered I did not have enough of it. The persisting nightmares and flashbacks were consuming much of my energy and I reached the point where I could hardly refresh myself between Friday evening and Monday morning. I also began to experience physical symptoms associated with stress.

We parted ways, and I knew I was in a serious personal crisis; I could no longer continue at the high stress level as before. Years back, I did a good job of rehabilitating my body, but my soul and psyche had remained wounded. For some four decades I had been able to compartmentalize and tuck away my emotional turmoil and lead a life as if the turmoil did not exist, but that had come to an end.

I had to deal with it if my future would be of any value. At age of fifty-six, I could still have a lot of life ahead of me. I finally realized I could not do everything on my own and needed help.

I took the leap and went to see a psychologist, something I had resisted doing in the past. I ended up seeing him twice a week for a whole year. It was the only thing I did, and it was the best investment of my life. I gained clarity and peace of mind, and that was priceless. It was the end of suffering with nightmares and fighting ghosts. I was discovering my true center and my spiritual self. I was now able to turn my painful past into a source of spiritual richness. I was now free to look at myself without barriers.

I was a very lucky man; not only did I miraculously survive the physical wounds of war, but I now survived the psychological crisis.

I have become keenly aware of the value of time and was determined not to waste it. For the past decades, my entire career had been focused on raising a family and creating an economic base; I had also been caught up in the endless chase to make more and more money, just for the sake of making it. Now I was able to see that our prudent investments could support us at an acceptable level, and I made the bold decision not to waste my life working just for the sake of making more money.

Avoiding stress and leading a healthy life had become paramount, so I decided to concentrate on activities that would nourish my soul, beginning with my love of classical music and black & white photography, extending to community service, giving back, "Tikun Olam" (repair of the world in Hebrew), or whatever else might come along. I was now a free man.

I havd become open to life's mysteries awaiting me. Life's next chapter was to begin without a plan, just following my nose. I was ready for more healing and spiritual experiences, wherever they would take me.

Magically, I did not have to wait very long.

IV.
THE REWARDS

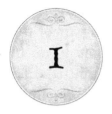

The New Beginning – Coming Out

In early 1988 we had houseguests from Israel, Rivka and Menachem, both from our old Daphna group. Menachem and I served in the same original Palmach squad in Daphna, and he also took part in the tragic battle for Nebbi Yusha; he was in the unit that attacked from the north and was lucky to have survived.

Our conversation turned to Nebbi Yusha; the annual memorial ceremony later that year would be special, commemorating the 40th anniversary of the battle. A major ceremony at the common gravesite was being planned with hundreds in attendance. The date was the 11th day of the Jewish month of Nissan, three days before Passover's first night. "Will you come?" they asked.

Almost instinctively I blurted out, "Of course I will," and after a short pause added, "and I would also like to deliver a eulogy as part of the ceremony." I didn't know where that came from, but I opened my big mouth and I was committed. Indeed, I was a new man following the year in counseling. I had a great deal of trepidation, but I was ready to deal with this painful subject. This was going to be my public coming-out, the peak of my healing journey.

Now I had to write the eulogy, in Hebrew. It was my single focus for the next two months prior to leaving for Israel, and it consumed my emotional and intellectual energies. I could no longer hold back; I had to put it all out. I was filled with excitement and anguish.

The question I struggled most with was: "What motivated us in the heat of battle to risk our lives in an attempt to rescue a comrade, knowing we most likely might lose our own doing it?"

After long and painful soul-searching, I concluded it was "love." Our bond was so powerful that the thought of leaving a comrade behind was totally unacceptable.

With this question resolved, I proceeded to write the eulogy.

This would be the first time since the battle forty years earlier that one of the battle's participants would speak at the annual memorial ceremony.

It was a beautiful clear day in the Galilee when I stood
by my brothers' grave and spoke. Here is the English
version:

It was in the still of the night, forty years ago,
    like lions we climbed this mountaintop,
hope in our hearts and the guns ready to go.
With your blood and death, my friends,
    you have consecrated this earth,
    and made us all into one...
blessed with the gift of love...
    known only to those who'd rather die
    than leave a friend behind!

And when the bullet hit my head -
    - it was all so quick!
for a moment I thought it was just a rock,
    or perhaps a mule's kick!
But instantly I was so helpless,
    floating and sinking into the dark abyss,
And I knew: Bullet ... head ... this is it!
    Surprise, it's almost painless!

And I wept within:
Too bad, still a virgin...so young!
"Farewell, Father, Mother, and friends...
And the air kept flowing out of my lungs…

And suddenly I was awake ...
yes, that was after eight days,
    glad and surprised to be alive;
But the voice has been haunting me ever since:
    "Why me and not them,
    why was it I who survived?"

And when I regained some speech and strength,
    I whispered slowly:
"How soon before I can go back to the field?"
And the doctor smiled,
                    bent over me and said:
    "For you, young man, the war is over,
    just be glad that you were not killed!"

Little did he know, this wonderful man,
that he left my heart broken, with deep, deep pain.

My soul is scarred, filled with doubts:
    I survived...
    I failed...
    I did not do enough!
Tell me, Mother, where did I go wrong,
    wasn't I supposed to be real tough?

It is here, in this presence, forty years later,
that I speak of my nightmares --
                    the unfinished battles-
'cause it was only you,
                    my friends who are still living,

who carried on the burden and horrors of doing more battles.

Today, in the presence of this grave,
I am expressing my gratitude and love
   to all those -- many I still don't know --
--who risked their lives to pull me out --
                       -- dead or alive.

And yes, my children, I am so proud to have been a part of the team on that fateful night,
Even if I were not so lucky...
...and remained asleep, never again to see light;
Because here, on that night, we were all made into one,
   blessed with the gift of love...known only to
                    those who'd rather die,
                 than leave a friend behind!

I stepped down from the podium into the arms of an old comrade; we hugged and cried together for a long time. A big, heavy burden was off my chest and I could breathe easy. No more secrets, no more sacred cows. I felt fully exposed and I was very comfortable with it.

I thought with the eulogy I had just experienced the peak of a long healing journey, but to my surprise that was just the gateway for more amazing things to come!

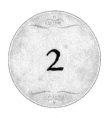

Ramot Naftali, 1988

While at the Nebbi Yusha memorial, I learned that two weeks hence, kibbutz Ramot Naftali, located one mile south of the fortress, would be celebrating its own 40th anniversary of breaking the Arab siege in the 1948 war.

Ramot Naftali was where I was carried to from the battlefield and remained for some 36 hours before being evacuated at night to the Hula valley below. I had been in a coma and had no memory of the event.

I decided I had a good reason to attend the celebration, although my own case played only a minute fraction of the total story there.

I arrived in the morning hours and found myself an uninvited anonymous visitor among several hundred attendees. We spent the morning hours touring the place and receiving presentations on key events that took place during the siege of the 1948 war. We then broke for an outdoors lunch in a park area.

Following lunch, we were treated to a program at the community hall staged by the local children.

Before closing the event, there was a surprise announcement from the stage, asking for the nine "babies" who were evacuated in the 1948 siege to come up to the stage and be recognized. Those were the babies evacuated by our unit that also carried me down the mountain. Nine men and women in their very early forties made their way to the stage to the audience's cheers and applause.

The announcer continued by asking if there was anybody in the audience who was among those who actually evacuated the babies to please come to the stage as well.

I realized at that moment I too belonged on the stage and boldly stepped forward.

Once up there, a microphone was passed around for us to identify ourselves. When I got it I simply said: "My name is Amnon Ben-Yehuda, I fought in the 1948 Nebbi Yusha battle, and--"

There was a commotion in the audience as two women were struggling to make their way to the stage. They rushed toward me, hugging me in amazement, as one grabbed the microphone and said excitedly, "The two of us were here forty years ago when they brought Amnon to us from the field and we took care of him while he was here. We had very little medical training and we had very little to treat him with; his head wound was very serious. All we could do was keep him from dehydration, so we kept his tongue and lips wet using a damp cloth, keeping turns around the clock between us. We never knew if Amnon survived the wounds. At times we placed inquiries on national radio but have had no response."

I was in shock and in heaven as the three of us were now standing on stage hugging and crying together, shedding tears of joy and happiness. Some in the audience came up and joined us.

After forty years, I miraculously found my angels who saved my life, Ruth and Malka, and they finally learned they actually did save a life. I was overwhelmed; I was levitating and overcome with emotions. We remained standing there for a long time, hugging, crying and kissing.

On my next visit to Israel the following year, I brought each one a gold necklace, the same as the one I have been wearing for many decades.

Ruth and her husband lived in a kibbutz in the Negev, and I was honored to be their houseguest.

Malka and her family lived in Jerusalem; she was a nurse at the Hadassah hospital. There again, I was honored to be their houseguest. On a quiet walk with her she shared with me that her own baby girl was among the nine infants to be evacuated in 1948 and how agonizing it was for her to hand her baby over to one of our brave Palmach warriors, to be evacuated. I also learned she had a younger son named Amnon.

Now I began the quest to identify all the brothers who carried me down the mountain or had any hand in my rescue. I had to poke and ask; nobody was coming forward willingly. The old code of silence was still prevalent, but ultimately I was successful.

3

Baruch Moskowitz

When I came to Israel in 1988 to deliver the eulogy at the 40th memorial anniversary, I was surprised and happy to see Baruch Moskowitz standing on the podium near me. We greeted each other warmly and made a date for me to visit him at his home in Tel-Aviv. His wife Sonia had passed on some years earlier and he was now living alone.

About eighty years of age, trim and with a sharp mind, he was a bitter man, still in mourning for his only son Malachi.

I must have symbolized to him something special--the one who miraculously survived the battle. I lent him an ear while he poured his heart out.

He told me a story about my father that I never knew before; the two had been business acquaintances.

The battle in 1948 took place on the night between Monday and Tuesday; the families of the fallen learned about their losses only through a newspaper story in the Friday-morning edition, listing the names of the fallen. I was brought to the hospital on Thursday evening or the same Friday morning and operated on. My parents spent much of that day at the hospital. Following the surgery, my doctor set my recovery odds at 0.5%.

This is what Baruch told me. "Did you know, Amnon, that your father came to our house on that Friday evening, straight from the hospital, to offer his condolences?"

"No," I said, "never knew about it, he never told me."

"Well, here is what your father said to me. 'Baruch, in a way I envy you, because you already know ... but we still do not know!' -- and he broke down crying."

I realized at that moment how my parents had done a good job of hiding their emotional agonies from me, or perhaps It was their way of trying to protect me.

As the afternoon was getting long and we began to conclude our conversation, he asked if I ever received a copy of the memorial book the twelve parents had published in memory for their fallen sons, members of the Daphna group.

"No," I replied, "I must have already been away at Berkeley at the time it was published."

He paused for a moment and said, "Just wait a minute." He stepped out to the adjoining room and after a while came back with a book in his hand.

"Amnon, this is my copy and I want you to have it."

I was stunned, speechless, and honored; it was a sacred moment and a sacred gift. Baruch was entrusting me with one of his most precious reminders of his fallen son.

We hugged and parted ways.

On my visit to Israel the following year, I rang him up. The line had been disconnected. I later learned Baruch had passed away.

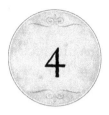

Back In San Diego

I was back home in San Diego from the most deeply moving and personally valuable trip to Israel. I had no plans to do any follow-up with it in San Diego or the USA in general -- I'd just savor it.

But reality was different, because I had set wheels in motion and there was no going back; events were beginning to happen on their own momentum.

After several weeks at home, I received a letter from Israel, from Menachem S., an old member of our Palmach Daphna group.

In the main he wrote:

"Dear Amnon, you may not remember me, but I was one of the guys who carried you down the mountain from kibbutz Ramot Naftali. Professionally I am a film producer, working for the Israel Educational TV Network.

"All my life I wanted to produce a documentary about the Nebbi Yusha battle but was unable to deal with subject due to my own guilt at not having participated in the battle itself.

"After hearing your eulogy a few weeks ago, and your expression of guilt of survival – **you, of all people**! -- my own guilt feelings have dissipated and I am now ready to do the documentary. I am planning to start filming at next year's memorial ceremony and I hope you will be there."

Of course I remembered Menachem; we met in Tel Aviv after I returned home from the hospital and he "damned" me for being so heavy on the stretcher.

And of course I was going to be there the following year.

I was settling back into my routine life in San Diego. At our San Diego Rotary Club's meeting I was greeted by Gary, our club president, with "Amnon, I have not seen you in a while, where have you been?" -- so I told him I'd been to Israel. "Well," he said, "I'd like to hear some more about it; how about breakfast?"

After listening to me over breakfast he asked, "How about telling this story to our Rotary club?"

I choked, but I had to accept; you do not refuse a request from the club's president. This would be my first time of giving a speech to our club with about 325 members in attendance. It would be the first time in the USA, apart from my immediate family, that I would talk about my wartime and healing experiences. It was not in my plans, but events were no longer under my control. I started the healing process, and it was now snowballing under its own momentum. I realized I had to learn to live with it, a part of my new me.

Several months later I made the presentation to our club. In about 20 minutes I managed to cover the story of my war experience, injury, loss of friends, miraculous survival, physical rehabilitation, successful career, my ghosts and stress effects, and resolution by going back to the common grave at the battle site to deliver the eulogy.

Giving the speech had a therapeutic effect on me, but at that time I still had no plan to do anything else with it. But again, I had no control over life's mysteries.

Several weeks after giving the talk at Rotary, I received a telephone call from a person introducing himself as the president of The Professional School of Psychological Studies in San Diego, saying he was a Rotarian member of another club and wished to meet with me. At the meeting he told me he happened to attend our Rotary club's meeting when I made the presentation and would like me to make a similar speech at the forthcoming graduation commencement ceremonies; the school would also award me with an honorary degree. I began to realize that things were serious and no longer under my control. I let go, and good things were just happening.

At the graduation ceremonies, I was surprised to see my co-recipient was Father Joe Carroll, the one person who has done so much for the homeless and the underprivileged in San Diego. Just standing on the same stage with Father Joe, a true giant, was more honorable for me than the honorary degree itself.

Like it or not, I now found myself on a speaking tour in the greater San Diego area; Rotary and other service clubs, various community groups, churches, and temples. I must have spoken several dozen times, and every time I did, I felt a bit more healed and spiritual.

The effects of military combat experience are unique and powerful, and now I saw it as a mission to share my experience with my audience. It's an experience that brings out the best and the worst in us. In combat we become killers, and at the same time are prepared to lose our own lives, even in a highly risky attempt, to save the life of a wounded comrade. We experience intense fear and learn to control and live with it. We create bonds with others, true brotherhood, one for all and all for one, with an intensity we never experience in ordinary life. And what do we do with all that when we return to routine civilian life, at home or on the job? It took me forty years to begin to open up and be able and willing to confront and talk about all this.

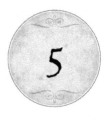

5

The Filming

I was back in Israel the following year for the annual memorial ceremonies at Nebbi Yusha, by the common grave site.

After the ceremony I was asked by Menachem, the film producer, to walk to the point where I was wounded. I could easily locate it; the ground has remained undisturbed and I remembered the crevices and small rocks in the ground. I was now standing literally on the spot where I took the bullet. The memories were powerful, and I was very emotional.

After the camera and crew were set, Menachem said, "Amnon, you have written and spoken about your guilt feelings; can you elaborate?"

I was not ready for this. I took a moment to collect my thoughts, and began:

"I left buddies here ... I did not complete my duty--"

"I was an NCO, I thought I was omnipotent, but 'he' took me before I took 'him,' a severe failure for me--"

"The fact that I survived, why me and not them ...
... as if I did not complete my assignment."

At that point, Menachem handed me a sheet of paper containing a poem and asked me to recite it out loud. It was a poem by Nathan Alterman, the great Israeli poet of the 1940s, covering the periods of the illegal immigration of Holocaust survivors from Europe and the 1948 War Of Independence.

I began reading:

"I will not forget this, my friend,
how you carried me on your back,
crawling valleys and mountains,

I will not forget
how you did not forsake me to die..."

I stopped reading, overwhelmed by the words that could have described my own experience. Both Menachem and I broke down, hugging and crying together. Menachem was one of the brothers who carried me down the mountain.

After we collected ourselves, he told me he'd had this poem posted over his desk at his office for decades, as a reminder of the amazing night they were able to carry me down the mountain. Hearing my eulogy a year earlier finally made it possible for him to broach the subject, and now he was finally making the documentary.

Here is the poem translated by me from Hebrew:

I will not forget this, my friend,
how you carried me on your back,
crawling mountains and valleys,

I will never forget
how you did not forsake me to die
when I hugged your neck,
like clinging to my own life.

It's night, my brother, put me down,
leave me here and run for your life
because my head is faint and my heart is pounding,
I shall not live to see the morning sun.

Promise me, when you visit my family,
tell them he was still a young man of wild ideas,
but he died being a real man.

By morning, my brother, I shall breathe no more,
but till morning, I shall never forget.

We stood there together crying and hugging, releasing tension that had been there for over forty years.

The poem has become my anthem. After returning home to San Diego, I superimposed the text on a photograph I had taken of the Nebbi Yusha fortress and distributed it among my old Daphna group comrades.

The Music

I was back in San Diego and the poem would not leave me. I was reciting it in my head morning, noon, and night. I was seeing it in my dreams. What a great poet Mr. Alterman was; my own English translation did not do justice to the linguistic beauty of the original Hebrew text. But primarily it was the story in the poem -- my God -- it could have been me. It was deeply personal.

I knew I had to do something important with it, but what?

Music! I decided to try to put the poem to music. I had never done that before, but I loved music and I played several instruments, so why not? But how to get started?

I spent time reading the poem over and over and

finally discovered the built-in rhythm of the text, and indeed it was all there. Next, I was sweating it out! I cannot describe how the tune finally came to me; I can only remember that it began with two measures in the middle with a unique theme that all of a sudden popped up, and from there it was developed to the entire poem. It was a long, exhausting, and arduous process with exciting results.

At one point, sitting at the piano during the composition process, my grandson asked, "Grandpa, why are you playing such sad music?" and I knew I was on the right track.

With a great deal of trepidation and a bit of chutzpah I decided to send the melody to Menachem in Israel who was putting the Nebbi Yusha documentary together. Playing the accordion, I recorded the melody into a tape recorder and called him.

"Hello Menachem, my dear friend, how are you?"

"Great, Amnon, and how about yourself?"

"Menachem, I have a surprise for you; I composed a melody to the poem 'I Will Not Forget This, My Friend,' and I want you to hear it."

"Fine, I am ready; put it on."

So I put the phone by the tape player and turned it on.

When the music was over, I picked up the phone and there was a long silence. Then I heard, "Amnon, you son of a bitch, you just made me make a complete change in the documentary. Please send me the music ASAP."

Hearing SOB from a good friend was a great compliment!

History was made. The documentary's title was changed to *I Will Not Forget This, My Friend* with the melody becoming its main musical theme.

Film Première

The next year I was back in Israel to watch the film's première. It would be broadcast on national television on the country's Memorial Day for the wars' dead.

I will be watching the film at Menachem's home, the film's producer and one of my rescuers.

The film manifested Menachem's lifelong ambition to produce a documentary on his trauma of the Nebbi Yusha battle disaster, and of the heroic acts of our brothers who lost their lives trying to save their wounded comrades. To him, I represented a redeeming aspect of the tragedy, with him having been a member of the team that managed to rescue me successfully. To him, I was also the catalyst who made it possible for him to overcome a forty-year period of suffering with guilt.

The two of us were brothers in so many ways!

The TV was on and we were anxiously waiting for the broadcast to begin. The sound of my music came first, and I became glued to the TV with stirred emotions. As the story unfolded, I was filled with painful memories. I was seeing pictures of brothers who were no longer with us and I was watching their mothers and other family members in their agonies. I was in a trance. The film went on for 42 minutes and most of the time my eyes were filled with tears. I felt numb, sad, happy, and proud.

I felt deeply how lucky I was to have survived the ordeal and recognized how much effort it took on the part of so many to make it happen. Could I ever repay them, and how? And why was I the one singled out to survive? I felt a sense of responsibility on my shoulders.

I knew I would need to view the film many more times before truly absorbing it, so I immediately made an effort to obtain a copy.

8

English Version

Back in San Diego, I was faced with the challenge of how to share this important documentary with my family and friends. Just like giving the talks about my Nebbi Yusha battle experience, showing the film to others could play a part in my own healing process. There was also a message in the film that must be shared with others.

The answer was obvious: Get it converted to English. How? Do it myself. I was already an Apple Mac user; all I needed was the special software and skill to use it. I purchased Final Cut Pro and spent exhausting weeks learning how to use it. I got the tape converted to a digital file, and my project began.

I had no idea what I was getting into! I quickly discovered that video editing was a huge time-consumer, but this was sacred work for me.

I ended up spending some three months doing the editing/conversion work, often working and crying at the same time. I was doing the language conversion on the fly, section by section, inserting English subtitles where a person was speaking to the camera in Hebrew. I paid attention to every nuance and made sure it was reflected in the translation. Two local friends provided the voice-over recordings for the two announcers in the film.

The emotional healing payoff for me was immense. Film editing required going over each and every video section repeatedly until I was satisfied with the results, so it seemed like I ended up viewing the film an endless number of times. Often, I would take a break because I was overwhelmed with emotions; I needed to calm myself down and seek my center. At times, I had to stop for the day. This was my existence for three full months and a powerful healing benefit, being forced to confront the deepest of feelings over and over.

The showings of the documentary have become an additional level in my healing process. I have shown it to Rotary and other service organizations, civic groups, temples, and churches. The film is always followed by a Q&A session that usually would give me the opportunity to dig deeper into the subject.

Early on I was reluctant to show the film to teenage groups, but I was proven wrong. I will never forget when following a viewing one high school student asked, "Were you not afraid?" This was a simple, innocent question that I never heard from an adult.

"Yes," I answered, "I was very much afraid, but we learned to control it. The worst fear I felt was before the first shot was fired; but after that I would function like a machine, and that took training."

What I did not say was that many years later, some of those paralyzing fearful moments would reappear to haunt me.

A direct link to the documentary is:

https://vimeo.com/76179028

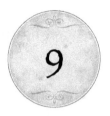

Mother

I believed I was reaching the point of emotional balance and peace of mind; my nightmares had disappeared. I was now feeling privileged and enriched by my life's journey and the healing I'd been through, beginning with my one year in psychotherapy and the eulogy I delivered for my fallen comrades in 1988 at the common gravesite.

Being filmed for the documentary while standing on the ground where I was shot was a powerful moment of truth and inner strength. It was further amplified by reading aloud, on camera, Nathan Alterman's great poem, which opened my gate of gratitude to all those who saved my life.

Putting the poem to music expressed the deepest level of emotions and pain from within me. I still feel the deep pain every time I hear or sing the tune.

I identified all and met with most of those who had a hand in saving my life. I have thanked them all and my music was in their honor.

I then realized there was one story I missed all along-- that of my parents. We never talked about this subject in the past.

Now that I myself was a grandfather, older than my parents were when I was wounded, for the first time I could ask myself how I would have felt if I were in their shoes, seeing a son mortally wounded?

My father had died years earlier. My mother was in her late eighties and living alone in Israel when I asked her, "Mom, can you tell me how you learned about my injury and what happened on that day?"

She thought for a moment and said, "It was on a Friday morning. Passover Seder would be celebrated on that evening. Dr. Mannheim came to the house on behalf of the Haganah to inform us you had been wounded in action and were being delivered to the Beilinson hospital near Tel-Aviv."

After a pause she continued, "Dad and I rushed to the hospital, where we were informed you were already in the preparation room for surgery."

She was now becoming agitated and said, "I wanted to see you at any cost before surgery, so I kept watch in the hallway between the preparation and surgery rooms. After a long wait, finally the door opened, and they were wheeling you out on a gurney. And do you know what happened?"

"No, Mom," I said.

"I lost control and I jumped at you crying out over and over -- Amnon, Amnon, this is your mother! And do you know what happened?" she asked.

I said, "No, Mother, I was in a coma."

With her voice trembling she said, "You slowly turned your head toward me and said, 'Mother, I love you.'"

I was stunned and moved to the core; she had kept this story to herself for over forty years!

I suddenly realized it was her way of trying to protect me all these years. With tears in my eyes I gave her a big hug and said, "Thank you, Mother. I know, I understand, and I love you--I love you very much!"

This was my truly healing moment.

PHOTOS

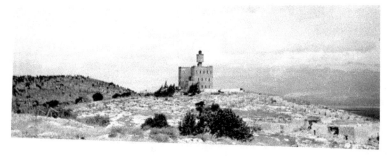

Nebbi Yusha fortress, taken in 1949,
from point where I was shot.

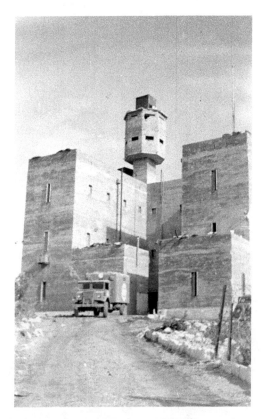

Nebbi Yusha fortress, close-up, 1949.

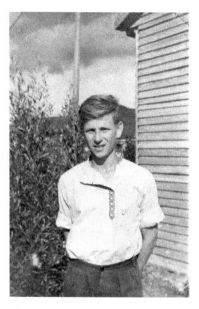

Amnon, in kibbutz Daphna, Palmach, 12/1947

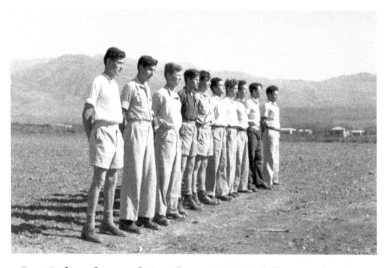

Our Palmach squad, Daphna, 1/1948, following battle in K'far Szold. Amnon is 3rd from left

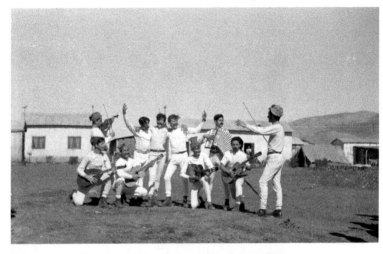

Our Palmach squad, Daphna, 12/1947, celebrating receipt of winter underwear. Amnon is 5th from right

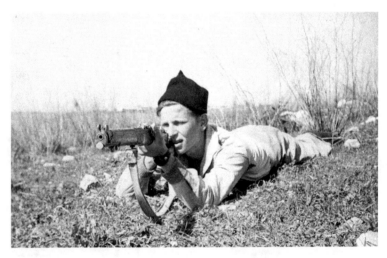

Amnon, in training

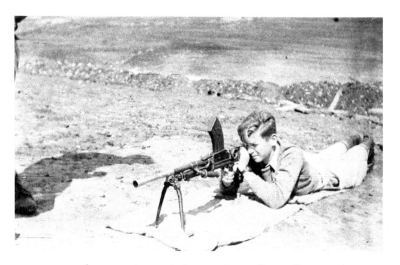

Amnon, in training, using a Bren Gun

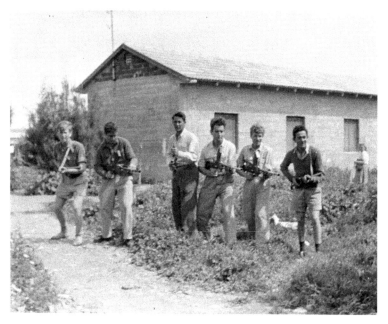

In Palmach first command course. Amnon is 1st from left

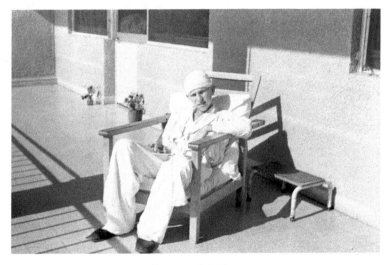

Amnon, in hospital following surgery

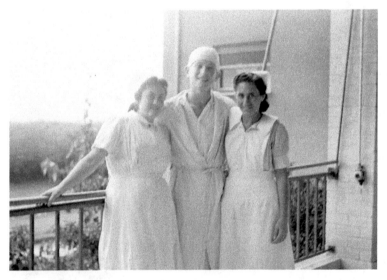

Amnon, in hospital, with nurses

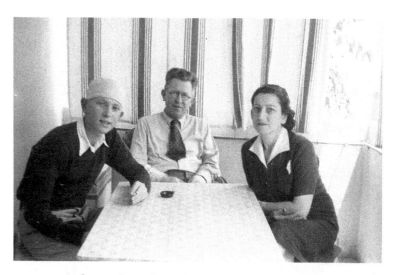

At home from hospital, with parents. 5/1947

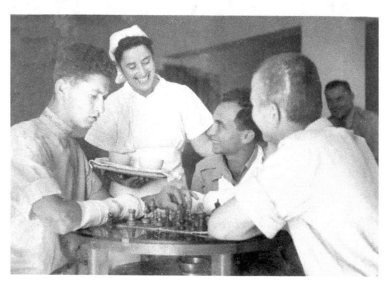

*Amnon, in convalescent center, with two other wounded
brothers from the Nebbi Yusha battle*

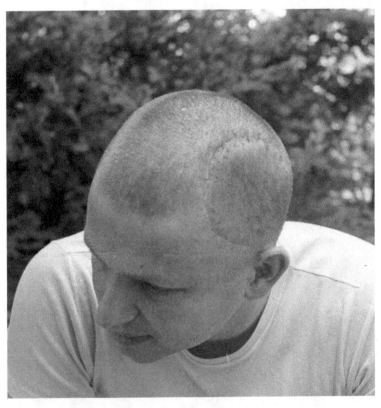

Detroit, 1954, following surgery, inserting a plastic plate

CPSIA information can be obtained
at www.ICGtesting.com
Printed in the USA
BVHW062320071022
648929BV00012B/1283